ISSUES in
NURSING

Readings selected from books
and periodicals to form a basis
for discussion of the problems
in nursing today

ISSUES in
NURSING

BONNIE BULLOUGH
VERN BULLOUGH
Editors

SPRINGER PUBLISHING COMPANY, Inc.
NEW YORK

PREFACE

American nursing is in the midst of revolutionary changes. Old ways of doing things are being challenged, modified, and discarded. Nursing has grown in complexity with the result that more is expected of the nurse. Some of these expectations are contradictory, and these contradictions have caused nursing to become a center of controversy. Nursing employment patterns have changed as institutional nursing has grown and private duty declined. The educational system is in a period of rapid growth in many directions. While these changes are interesting to observe, they are also somewhat bewildering.

In this book we have attempted to provide some answers, both as to why the changes have occurred and what the future holds for nursing. We have not given any simple answers because anyone who attempts to chart the future for nursing will find that there *are* none. Some nurses will prefer one path while others will choose different ones. To allow the nurse to make as intelligent a decision as possible, we have gathered many different proposals and analyses of the issues in nursing. Although we admit to having certain biases, such as favoring better salaries and working conditions for nurses, we have tried to avoid advocating any one particular point of view to the exclusion of others.

Before proposed paths can be understood, some of the past decisions which have affected nursing have to be examined; to this end we have included some material from the recent past. We have extracted articles from many different sources, representing various styles of writing. Longer selections have been considerably edited so that the material would fit into the book. Our only purpose in editing was to present the concepts of the authors more concisely and not to change their words. Many of the articles are not by nurses and we have not included many of the great names in the history of nursing in order to present as varied a viewpoint as possible and to avoid overlapping. Nurse authors are indicated by "R.N." after their names in the Table of Contents.

We have chosen five topics which are central to the future of nursing and over which there is considerable disagreement: nursing education, professionalization, the nursing role, economic issues, and changing aspects of patient care. Obviously this leaves many problem areas without discussion, but the organization of the material is broad enough to include more than might at first be evident. We deliberately excluded a discussion of the economic needs of the patients, a major area of nursing concern, because we felt that such material would be outmoded by the operation of Medicare, the evaluation of which will take several years.

Each section of the book is meant to be read independently although a better understanding of the problems facing nurses can be had by reading the whole book. Some articles and topics supplement others. Each section opens with a brief exposition of the issues; then some historical materials are presented, and this is followed by a discussion of current trends from various points of view. Not all articles in the book reflect our own view nor even that of the majority of nurses, but our purpose in including them is to provide a basis for opinion formation. The book is directed at three general categories of readers: students who want to know the issues in nursing, teachers who might want to use the book as a text or as supplemental reading, and nurses who want a better understanding of the current issues in their profession. This last group is a rapidly growing one as nurses realize that education for nursing is a continuing process and not merely something which was completed at their graduation. The constant expansion of scientific and technological knowledge is making new demands on nurses, and the only possible way to meet these demands is through some form of continuing education, either self-initiated or in organized programs.

We hope that nurses will be better informed about the issues in nursing after reading the book and that it will assist them in effectively planning for the future.

JUNE 1966

The Editors

BONNIE BULLOUGH, R. N., M.S., *Research Assistant, U.C.L.A.*

VERN BULLOUGH, Ph.D., *Professor of History, San Fernando Valley State College, Northridge, California, and Lecturer, California College of Medicine of the University of California.*

CONTENTS

ACKNOWLEDGEMENTS

Permission to reprint the selections in this book, granted by the following publishing houses, journals, and organizations, is hereby gratefully acknowledged:

G. P. Putnam's Sons
McGraw-Hill Book Company
Nursing Outlook
RN Magazine
American Journal of Nursing
Nursing Research
The Reporter
Journal of Social Issues
The Carnegie Foundation for the Advancement of Teaching
Russell Sage Foundation
Institute of Industrial Relations, U.C.L.A.
American Nurses' Association
National League for Nursing, Inc.
U.S. Department of Health, Education and Welfare
U.S. Department of Labor, Bureau of Labor Statistics

THE EDUCATION OF NURSES

Modern nursing, at least in the minds of its founders, was distinguished from earlier forms of nursing primarily because of its training programs. Training schools proved to be such an advantage to the hospitals in cutting down the costs of nursing care yet improving its quality that schools were established rapidly in a vast number of hospitals. Unfortunately, many of them were unsuited for the training of nurses, and the quality of education they offered was poor. Some sort of educational reform was necessary but achieving it was no easy task—and reform is still going on. The first step was to improve the hospital schools, and this is where the early leaders of nursing concentrated their efforts. One of the most influential was Mary Adelaide Nutting, a dominant figure in American nursing.

1.
Some Problems of Training Schools for Nurses

by Mary Adelaide Nutting

It is when we approach the actual education of our student and attempt to carry out the promises which have been made to her, that the resisting power of the hospital becomes more and more strongly felt, and the enormous difficulty with which it meets even the least of its obligations in this respect is clearly seen. There is no place in its strenuous scheme of life for the machinery of a school. All the space, the effort, the means which the hospital can provide are needed to carry out its immediate purpose, which is the care of the sick, and any scheme of education must, of necessity, take a sec-

---

From an address given before the American Hospital Association in Toronto, Canada in 1908, and later reprinted in *A Sound Economic Basis for Schools of Nursing*. New York: G. P. Putnam's Sons, 1926, pp.18-39, *passim*. It is worthy of note that Miss Nutting found the same problems to exist in 1926 that she did in 1908, and did not modify her original remarks.

ondary and insignificant place. A school, to fulfil its functions, cannot take such a place; it calls for teachers, class-rooms, equipment, and every subject offered in the curriculum needs these to a greater or less degree. Some subjects, to be taught at all, require a laboratory as well. The teacher is presumably a person especially prepared to teach, with ability to handle certain subjects adequately, and with time to meet her class regularly, to know her students, and to be interested in their advancement.

How far is it possible for the hospital to provide anything of this nature? In most of the thousand schools of nursing a good proportion of the instruction provided is that comprised in a series of lectures, given gratuitously by different physicians of the staff. That they are frequently cheerfully given, and that much of such teaching is excellent, as far as it goes is true, but this does not essentially alter the main facts, which are that such teaching is dependent in its character upon the particular views of that particular physician as to the education of nurses, and upon his good will and circumstances as to regularity and system. It has no stable character of its own. It may or may not cover a certain definite ground. It may be good, or it may be worthless as teaching. The school has little power to choose which it shall be. With neither means to pay for suitable teaching, nor freedom to choose the teacher, it must accept whatever is within its reach. I have known an entire short course of lectures, of great importance, offered in the curriculum of a school by a talented, but busy, physician, postponed from month to month, and finally the year concluded without even one lecture having been given. I have known the opening lecture of a course postponed for four weeks in succession because the physician giving the course was either suddenly called out of town, or engaged by an emergency or by an important dinner. I have known certain subjects which belonged to the very beginning of the year transferred to the end of it, or even to a subsequent year to suit the convenience of the lecturer and yet upon these lectures at a given time might depend the ability of a whole group of students to comprehend much of the practical work they were then engaged in performing. In hospitals where there is a medical school attached, there is less difficulty in securing systematic teaching, since the embryo professor of medicine is apt to look upon the school as a useful place in which to test his own powers. The teaching thus given by young residents is often good as to substance, and is sometimes carried on with interest, occasionally with enthusiasm, but much of it bears the hall-marks of youth and inexperience.

Turning from the teacher to the subjects taught, this matter also is governed by the ability or will of the hospital to provide. Such a fundamental subject in nursing as foods, their properties, preparation and uses, was not taught in many schools in certain States until laws of the State for the registration of nurses made it necessary for the hospital with which they were connected, to provide this most essential teaching; and there are other important subjects, equally fundamental, which may be entirely omitted from the training school curriculum. Although the instruction in most of our schools is elementary from beginning to end, the hospital has full power to restrict this teaching in various ways; it may reduce the ground covered in a certain subject to the barest outline. This power rests with the hospital, and at times it may really rest with one member of the Board of Trustees or the hospital staff. The individual who thinks "this idea of teaching nurses so much is all nonsense, anyway," will not view with favor anything which carries the pupil nurse very far from her long hours of practical work in the wards, and he will be especially suspicious, and apt to shy violently at the mention of bacteriology, for instance, or the still more dangerous subject of pathology. Yet, in my opinion, there is no one subject in which it is essential for the nurse to be more solidly and thoroughly grounded than in bacteriology. Dealing with the causes of disease and with their prevention, it forms the very basis on which her subsequent training and education and her safety and efficiency in her professional work must rest. The subject, in fact, in certain of its essentials, might well form part of the education of every citizen, and it is interesting to note that while on the one hand there may be anxious discussion in schools of nursing as to whether it is advisable to give the student nurses four or six lectures on this subject, in another direction, students of domestic science who are preparing to teach cookery to children in the public schools are required to have, and rightly, a full half-year course of 60 hours in bacteriology.

As to class-rooms and equipment, while in certain schools there is one class-room and some equipment, in hundreds of schools there is not the slightest pretence of either. The class-room may be the screened-off end of a sitting room; it may be the dining room; it may be any room which can at short notice be supplied with chairs and table and blackboard. In scarcely any school is there a class-room large enough for the entire body of pupils to be assembled together; and when we come to equipment, material for teaching, such as microscopes, maps, charts, photographs, models and specimens, there is such a painful void that one sometimes wonders how teaching can be carried on at all.

It is, I think, generally conceded that teaching given in the evening, after a day of hard physical effort, is of very limited value. Yet, until recently, nearly all of the teaching in training schools was given in the evening, and the eight o'clock lecture was the educational event of the week. I am happy to say that there is now a distinct effort being made to bring classes and lectures forward into the afternoon.

As to the practical instruction and training in the wards, it will probably be said that here at least the hospital provides amply for all needs of the student, for even at the minimum she must work in the wards or other hospital departments eight hours daily; so that, while two hours weekly is the average, and three the maximum for theoretical teaching except in preliminary courses, from fifty to sixty hours of ward work are required weekly of the student, even under the easiest conditions. The suggestion that in any of our training schools for nurses there is an undue proportion of theory would be ridiculous, if it were not pathetic. Most of us are mentally lazy, and it is often true that the students will say they love their active work in the wards, and do not enjoy their studies; but that does not alter the fact that they need to study, whether they enjoy it or not. It is probable that if they were less physically tired, studying would seem more attractive.

But how about this teaching and training in the ward, which we have agreed is so valuable? If it is so all-important, it is, of course, carefully carried on by highly qualified nurses, specially prepared to teach over the patient the most skilled and perfect methods of nursing. The young student must be taught how to observe and record every trifling change in the patient's condition, and what action such a change calls for. She must be taught every process needed, in its every detail, and these processes are many. She must then practise each process assiduously, under criticism and supervision, until it can be performed with that ease which is the final perfection of skill; and then she must be taught further under what conditions the process itself must be varied, adjusted, modified to suit the different temperaments and needs of the sick.

Now, I do not need to say that anything even faintly resembling such a method of teaching is not carried out in any satisfactory way in any of our training schools. The student is in the ward to do the work, and to do as much as she can possibly accomplish in a given time. In many hospitals, especially in certain departments, she works under pressure every hour; and not only has she no time to be taught, but the head nurse of the ward has no time to teach her. This, I think, is true of all large general hospitals, where there is an acute service. It is specially true of those with medical schools attached, where, for clinical purposes, prolonged and repeated rounds may almost detach the head nurse entirely from her ward. As Superintendent of Nurses, I have many times been unable to secure a needed conversation with a head nurse for an entire morning, and have gone to a certain ward as many as four times between the hours of eight and twelve, to find her each time in attendance upon a clinic. In such hospitals there are usually one or more assistants who could render valuable service in the way of bed-side teaching, but their executive duties are many, and they can seldom do even a fraction of what is needed in this direction.

In smaller hospitals such opportunities would be better, that is, the head nurse might have more time, but here again one is met by the fact that there is often no head nurse in a ward but merely a student at the helm, and also that the limitation in numbers and variety of patients are such as to greatly restrict the field for teaching. In certain small hospitals all of the teaching in both class-room and ward is done by the overworked executive head of the hospital. So that this invaluable field of teaching, the hospital ward with its groups of patients becomes the place where the student passes through a succession of similar experiences and performs over and over again certain acts; but it is not used as it might be for definite study of disease, for observation, careful instruction and suitable development in nursing knowledge and skill. The best actual teaching then is that given in order, system and discipline. "A nurse may potter about in a ward for a year and learn very little without definitely directed teaching," said Florence Nightingale many years ago.

It needs no argument of mine, I am sure, to convince you that the preparation for any of the various kinds of work which have been touched upon here needs to be sound, thorough and carefully planned, and that no brief or limited preparation will suffice. In saying, however, that it cannot be given in less than three years, I would not be understood as agreeing that a course of such length should be offered in the majority of hospitals. Unless a hospital can provide for a full training in the main services, it is not justified in keeping the student for three years, and the tendency in hospitals and sanitaria with very limited opportunities to insist upon a three years' training, must be looked upon as deplorable. Looked at baldly, one sees the institution willing to require an additional year of work from the student, in return for which it can offer little she actually needs. I have in mind a private hospital, the property of one man, in which the work is, I believe, largely surgical. A training school with a two years' course was established, and not long since a third year was added. Almost all of the special nursing in this hospital is done by the students, and I am told they are placed on special duty at a very early stage in their training. One year of training would probably amply cover all that this enterprising institution has to offer.

In this attempt to place before you some, at least, of the problems with which the training school for nurses is confronted, I am led to believe that they are all mere aspects and phases of one single problem, and that problem is the relation of the hospital to the training school.

Familiar as we all are with the present system, it is not easy to entertain the idea of anything different. Yet there are those who feel that, in the best interests of both hospital and training school, some reconstruction of that system is necessary; that much of the teaching, especially all of that fundamental work included in the preparatory course now given in the hospital, should be given outside of it, in a central school, which could do for a number of hospitals what each one is now trying inadequately to do for itself; and that this central school should take upon itself the full direction of the education of the student and the responsibility of arranging with different hospitals for her practical training in all the various services. In other words, that the school of nursing should rest upon a separate foundation not unlike that of the medical school. Such central schools could, in course of time, help to solve the problem of nursing in some of the small and special hospitals, now struggling to maintain their own separate schools. I should like to add my personal belief that the pupil should pay for her training straight through, and that she should be far more independent of the requirements of the hospital, which, in some departments, should be partly met by salaried workers.

I am by no means presenting new ideas to you in these suggestions. Some of them have already been made by a good many people. The need of such a central school was admirably presented by Dr. Francis Denny in the *Boston Medical and Surgical Journal* for June, 1903; Dr. Richard Cabot has written frequently and convincingly on the subject; while Mrs. Hunter Robb, in a noteworthy paper read in Washington some years ago, suggested the main conditions for such a school, which should be carefully studied. An article by Dr. Oldfield in the *Westminster Review,* a few years ago, advocated a Royal College of Nurses and the granting of degrees. I confess that nursing, as I see it, seems to me as worthy of a place in the scheme of the university as any art or science in it.

I have tried in this paper to lay before you as faithfully as I could some of the difficulties with which our training schools are contending, difficulties which are apparently the inevitable result of the present relationship between school and hospital. To me, at least, they seem serious, and I believe they merit your most thoughtful consideration. This is no question of doctor versus nurse, or of hospital versus training school; each is essential in the work of the other. The question is, what is the very best that we can do for our training schools for nurses? The various classes of people and the institutions in the community which have come to lean upon the trained nurse, and to be dependent upon her services, require of us that we should, in our teaching and training, put her in the way of developing those services to their full power and usefulness.

One of the reasons why the hospital training school was so well established in nursing was that this was the normal method of training all "medical" practitioners, including physicians. Before nurses could begin to break away from the dominance of the hospitals and maintain schools whose prime interest was in the education of nurses, it was necessary for someone to undertake basic reforms in medical education. The prime movers in this direction were Abraham Flexner and the Carnegie Foundation for the Advancement of Teaching. The following extract is from a report which led to fundamental reforms in medical education. Notice the similarity between the complaints of Flexner and those of Adelaide Nutting.

2.
Medical Education in the United States

by Abraham Flexner

The striking and significant facts which are here brought out are of enormous consequence not only to the medical practitioner, but to every citizen of the United States and Canada; for it is a singular fact that the organization of medical education in this country has hitherto been such as not only to commercialize the process of education itself, but also to obscure in the minds of the public any discrimination between the well trained physician and the physician who has had no adequate training whatsoever. As a rule, Americans, when they avail themselves of the services of a physician, make only the slightest inquiry as to what his previous training and preparation have been. One of the problems of the future is to educate the public itself to appreciate the fact that very seldom, under existing conditions, does a patient receive the best aid which it is possible to give him in the present state of medicine, and that this is due mainly to the fact that a vast army of men is admitted to the practice of medicine who are untrained in sciences fundamental to the profession and quite without a sufficient experience with disease. A right education of public opinion is one of the problems of future medical education.

The significant facts revealed by this study are these:

1. For twenty-five years past there has been an enormous over-production

From *Medical Education in the United States and Canada*. New York: The Carnegie Foundation, 1910, pp. x–xi.

of uneducated and ill trained medical practitioners. This has been in absolute disregard of the public welfare and without any serious thought of the interests of the public. Taking the United States as a whole, physicians are four or five times as numerous in proportion to population as in older countries like Germany.

2. Over-production of ill trained men is due in the main to the existence of a very large number of commercial schools, sustained in many cases by advertising methods through which a mass of unprepared youth is drawn out of industrial occupations into the study of medicine.

3. Until recently the conduct of a medical school was a profitable business, for the methods of instruction were mainly didactic. As the need for laboratories has become more keenly felt, the expenses of an efficient medical school have been greatly increased. The inadequacy of many of these schools may be judged from the fact that nearly half of all our medical schools have incomes below $10,000, and these incomes determine the quality of instruction that they can and do offer.

Colleges and universities have in large measure failed in the past twenty-five years to appreciate the great advance in medical education and the increased cost of teaching it along modern lines. Many universities desirous of apparent educational completeness have annexed medical schools without making themselves responsible either for the standards of the professional schools or for their support.

4. The existence of many of these unnecessary and inadequate medical schools has been defended by the argument that a poor medical school is justified in the interest of the poor boy. It is clear that the poor boy has no right to go into any profession for which he is not willing to obtain adequate preparation; but the facts set forth in this report make it evident that this argument is insincere, and that the excuse which has hitherto been put forward in the name of the poor boy is in reality an argument in behalf of the poor medical school.

5. A hospital under complete educational control is as necessary to a medical school as is a laboratory of chemistry or pathology. High grade teaching within a hospital introduces a most wholesome and beneficial influence into its routine. Trustees of hospitals, public and private, should therefore go to the limit of their authority in opening hospital wards to teaching, provided only that the universities secure sufficient funds on their side to employ as teachers men who are devoted to clinical science.

In view of these facts, progress for the future would seem to require a very much smaller number of medical schools, better equipped and better conducted than our schools now as a rule are; and the needs of the public would equally require that we have fewer physicians graduated each year, but that these should be better educated and better trained. With this idea accepted, it necessarily follows that the medical school will, if rightly conducted, articulate not only with the university, but with the general system of education. Just what form that articulation must take will vary in the immediate future in different parts of the country. Throughout the eastern and central states the movement under which the medical school articulates with the second year of the college has already gained such impetus that it can be regarded as practically accepted. In the southern states for the present it would seem that articulation with the four-year high school would be a reasonable starting-point for the future. In time the development of secondary education in the south and the growth of the colleges will make it possible for southern medical schools to accept the two-year college basis of preparation. With reasonable prophecy the time is not far distant when, with fair respect for the interests of the public and the need for physicians, the articulation of the medical school with the university may be the same throughout the entire country. For in the future the college or the university which accepts a medical school must make itself responsible for university standards in the medical school and for adequate support for medical education. The day has gone by when any university can retain the respect of educated men, or when it can fulfill its duty to education, by retaining a low grade professional school for the sake of its own institutional completeness.

The first major reforms in nursing education in the United States came as a result of a report by Josephine Goldmark, who carried out a study under the auspices of the Committee for the Study of Nursing Education. This committee had been appointed by the Rockefeller Foundation in January, 1919, to conduct a study of "the proper training of public health nurses." It soon became apparent that training in this one area could not be separated from the overall problem of nursing education, and the scope of the inquiry was broadened to include "a study of general nursing education, with a view to developing a program for further study and for recommendation of further procedures."

3.

Nursing Education in the 1920's

by Josephine Goldmark and the Committee for the
Study of Nursing Education

The development of the hospital training school for nurses constitutes a unique chapter in the history of education. In almost all fields of professional life education has begun on a basis of apprentice training. The first law schools and the first medical schools were the outgrowth of the lawyer's and the physician's office. In nearly all other fields than that of nursing, however, even in such relatively new professions as journalism and business advertising, education has outgrown the apprentice stage and leadership has passed into the hands of independent institutions, organized and endowed for a specifically educational purpose. The training of nurses, on the other hand, is still in the main, actually if not technically, directed by organizations created and maintained for the care of disease, rather than for professional education.

The progress which has been accomplished in nursing education, under such anomalous conditions, is such as to reflect high credit upon both hospital administrators and the leaders of the nursing profession. The hospitals have in many instances been inspired by a broad and constructive vision of training school possibilities; while the devotion with which nursing directors have labored for high standards, often against almost insuperable obstacles, calls for the warmest admiration. Yet the conflict of interests between a policy of hospital administration, which properly aims to care for the sick at a minimum cost, and a policy of nursing education which with equal propriety aims to concentrate a maximum of rewarding training into a minimum time, is a real and vital one.

The fact that a field so tempting as that of modern nursing, with its remarkable possibilities of service in public health, in institutional management, and in teaching, fails to attract students in the number, and of the quality, we should desire strongly suggests that there is some shortcoming in the established avenues of approach to the nursing profession. The hospitals themselves, depending as they do so largely upon student nurses for their routine operation, have in past years found themselves seriously handicapped by the small number of applicants, and many a superintendent will testify to the fact that the difficulty of securing a high quality of nursing is one of the gravest which he has to meet. The phenomenally rapid growth

From *Nursing and Nursing Education in the United States*. New York: The Macmillan Company, 1923, pp. 17–26.

in the number of hospitals has created within a brief period a demand for a large number of students and the requirements for admission have therefore been kept at a very low level, thus resulting in a reduction in the proportion of well-educated applicants. For the good of the hospital, as well as for that of the nursing profession and of the public at large, a careful and dispassionate appraisal of the adequacy of the present day training school would seem to be urgently desirable.

Conditions Revealed by a Study of Typical Hospital Training Schools

An extensive survey of the vast field of hospital training schools (there are over 1,800 such schools in the United States) was obviously beyond the possible resources of our Committee. It was therefore decided to select a small group of schools, of reasonably typical character, for intensive study. Twenty-three such schools were finally chosen, representing large and small, public and private, general and special hospitals, in various sections of the United States. These schools were undoubtedly well above the median grade and their average may, we believe, be taken as fairly representative of the best current practice in nursing education. Each school was studied in detail by two types of investigators, one a practical expert in nursing education, and the other an experienced educator from outside the nursing field. By this means we aimed, on the one hand to secure competent criticism of nursing procedures, and on the other a broad view of general educational standards. The detailed results of this investigation as presented in Miss Goldmark's report, will, we believe, prove highly enlightening to the student of this problem.

The training of the nurse involves a certain basic knowledge of the fundamental chemical and biological sciences, theoretical instruction in the principles of nursing and, above all, supervised practical training in actual nursing procedures. In all three phases of this work Miss Goldmark's report reveals conspicuous successes and equally conspicuous failures; and the remarkable thing is that successes and failures so often appear side by side in the same institution.

Thus, we may find in a training school with a good ward service that the fundamental science courses fail because of wholly inadequate laboratory equipment. In another school, the theoretical instructor may show a hopeless lack of teaching ability (as in the case of class presentation which consisted in the dictation of questions and answers from a prehistoric notebook); or she may be so handicapped by other duties as to leave no time for the proper conduct of her classes. Lectures by physicians may be informative and inspiring in one department of a hospital; irregular in delivery, careless and dull in content, in another. Ward assignments are in many cases largely dictated by the need for hospital service rather than by the educational requirements of the students. This is clearly evidenced by the astonishing irregularity of the time spent on different services by individual students and by the marked deviation between all the time assignments actually performed and those scheduled in the official program of the course. Thus in one school where 7½ months were assigned to surgical service the members of a single class had actually worked on this service for from 7 to 13¾ months. Of the 23 schools surveyed by us one made no adequate provision for obstetrical service, while 5 gave no training in pediatrics, 7 no experience in communicable disease and 18 none in mental disease. In view of the difficulties in making affiliations in some of these subjects, notably in communicable and mental diseases, some of these omissions are scarcely to be wondered at.

The supervision of work on the wards was in certain instances notably inadequate. In only a few brilliantly exceptional cases was the ward work purposefully correlated with theoretical instruction. The lack of an intelligently planned progressive training was obvious in a large number of the hospitals studied, first year students often being found in positions of responsibility for which they were wholly unprepared, while seniors in another ward were repeating an educationally idle and profitless routine. Most striking of all, was the factor of time wasted in procedures, essential to the conduct of the hospital, but of no educational value to the student concerned. Hours and days spent in performing the work of a ward maid, in putting away linen, in sterilizing apparatus, in mending rubber gloves, in running errands, long after any important technique involved had become second nature, accounted in one typical hospital operating under the 8-hour system, where this problem was specially studied, for a clear wastage of between one-fourth and one-fifth of the student's working day.

The total amount of time assigned to ward service under the conditions which obtain in many hospitals is, in itself, a fairly complete obstacle to educational achievement. Our selected group of hospitals, surely in this respect far above the general average, shows a median day of between 8 and 8.5 hours on ward duty alone, exclusive of all classroom instruction. Irregular and excessive and unproductive night duty is the rule rather than the exception. Crowded and unattractive living conditions tend, in certain hospitals, to impair the morale of the student body; and an atmosphere of autocratic discipline frequently prevents the development of a psychological atmosphere favorable to effective co-operative effort.

The foregoing paragraphs present, we are aware, a somewhat gloomy picture. In presenting them, we would emphasize two points which are of major importance. In the first place, such shortcomings as have been pointed out are not fairly chargeable to deliberate neglect on the part of hospital authorities or nursing superintendents. In so far as they exist, they are due to the inherent difficulty of adjusting the conflicting claims of hospital management and nursing education, under a system in which nursing education is provided with no independent financial endowment for its specific ends. The difficulties involved in the task of resolving this conflict are perhaps illustrated by the fact that out of 144 registered training schools in New York State, 60 changed superintendents during a single recent year.

In the second place it is encouraging to note, by reference to Miss Goldmark's report, that every one of the shortcomings in hospital training discussed above has been corrected, with substantially complete success, in one or more of the training schools studied by our investigators. The difficulties are not insuperable. Each of them has been overcome in some schools and most of them in some of the best schools. Training schools exist today in which the student receives a sound and an inspiring education, with a minimum of sacrifice to the exigencies of hospital administration. Yet such schools are still the exception; and we are convinced that the progress we desire can come only through a frank facing of the truth. The following statement is, we believe, thoroughly justified by such facts as we have been able to obtain:

Conclusion. That, while training schools for nurses have made remarkable progress, and while the best schools of today in many respects reach a high level of educational attainment, the average hospital training school is not organized on such a basis as to conform to the standards accepted in other educational fields; that the instruction in such schools is frequently casual and uncorrelated; that the educational needs and the health and strength of students are frequently sacrificed to practical hospital exigencies; that such shortcomings are primarily due to the lack of independent endowments for nursing education; that existing educational facilities are on the whole, in the majority of schools, inadequate for the preparation of the high grade of nurses required for the care of serious illness, and for service in the fields of public health nursing and nursing education; and that one of the chief reasons for the lack of sufficient recruits, of a high type, to meet such needs lies precisely in the fact that the average hospital training school does not offer a sufficiently attractive avenue of entrance to this field.

Recommendations for the Improvement of the Hospital
Training School

Miss Goldmark's study has not stopped short with a revelation of the defects which are commonly found in the conduct of nursing education. It makes clear that only the co-ordination and standardization of the best existing practice is necessary in order to place nursing education on the plane where it belongs.

In the first place we believe that a training school which aims to educate nurses capable of caring for acute disease or of going on into public health nursing or supervisory and teaching positions, must require for entrance the completion of a high school course or its equivalent. Nearly one-third of all the training schools in the United States now make this requirement; and with 150,000 girls graduating from high schools every year it should be possible for well-organized courses to attract an ample number of candidates.

The course should begin with a preliminary term of 4 months' training in the basic sciences and in elementary nursing procedures with appropriate ward practice but without regular ward service, as outlined in Miss Goldmark's report. The necessary teaching personnel and laboratory equipment for the former may in many instances be secured by the smaller hospitals through the establishment of a central training course or by co-operation with high schools, normal schools, or junior colleges.

There should then follow a period of 24 months (including 2 months for vacation) devoted to a carefully graded and progressive course in the theory and practice of nursing, with lectures and ward practice so correlated as to facilitate intelligent case study and with the elimination of routine duties of no educational value. Hospital and dispensary services in medicine, surgery, pediatrics, obstetrics, communicable diseases and mental diseases should be provided through appropriate affiliation. Teachers and equipment should be of such a grade as would be acceptable in a reputable college or normal school.

We regard it as fundamental that the working day for the student nurse, including ward work and classroom periods, should not exceed 8 hours. The working week should not exceed 48 hours and preferably 44 hours. Training school experience, as well as a comparison with that accumulated in other educational fields, makes it clear that a longer period of scheduled work for the student is incompatible, either with educational attainment or with the maintenance of health.

By such an organization of the course of study, and particularly by the elimination of unrewarding routine service, we are convinced that the period of training may be safely shortened from the present standard of 3 years to 28 months. Such a saving would mean an increase of over 20 per cent in the potential output of the training school through the saving of time alone. The shortening of the course would, in itself, prove an attraction to the prospective student; but the main consideration to be kept in view is that the shorter course projected would not imply a lowering but a raising of educational standards. Miss Goldmark's analysis of the situation makes it clear that the intensively-planned course of 28 months would involve no substantial sacrifice in a single service as compared with the actual median practice of the present day, and would supply other services now almost universally neglected. It is the experience in every other field of education that the way to attract students is to raise standards, not to lower them. In medicine, in law, in engineering, in teaching, the schools which raise requirements are the ones from which students must be turned away; and even in nursing the success of the better schools furnishes convincing testimony to the same basic principle. It is the higher standing of the course here outlined, quite as much as its lessened length, which we are confident would insure an increase in the number of students, as well as an improvement in their quality.

There are, we believe, two fundamental essentials to the success of a training school planned on the suggested lines. It must first of all be directed by a board or a committee, organized more or less independently for the primary purposes of education. The interests of hospital management and of educational policy must necessarily at times conflict, and unless the educational viewpoint is competently represented the training school will infallibly suffer in the end. In the second place it is fundamental to the success of nursing education that adequate funds should be available for the educational expenses of the school itself, and for the replacement of student nurses by graduate nurses and hospital help in the execution of routine duties of a non-educational character. A satisfactory relationship between school and hospital demands careful cost-accounting and a clear analysis of the money value of services rendered by the school to the pupil and the hospital, by the pupil to the hospital, and by the hospital to the pupil and the school. The cost of adequate education must in any case be a paramount consideration, to which we shall return in a succeeding paragraph. Assuming its essential importance, the following conclusion seems to us justified:

Conclusion. That, with the necessary financial support and under a separate board or training school committee, organized primarily for educational purposes, it is possible, with completion of a high school course or its equivalent as a prerequisite, to reduce the fundamental period of hospital training to 28 months, and at the same time, by eliminating unessential, non-educational routine, and adopting the principles laid down in Miss Goldmark's report, to organize the course along intensive and co-ordinated lines with such modifications as may be necessary for practical application; and that courses of this standard would be reasonably certain to attract students of high quality in increasing numbers.

Postgraduate Nursing Education

The course of 28 months discussed above would furnish the complete education for a student desiring to practice as a bedside nurse in private duty or in hospitals and other institutions; and its completion should entitle her to the diploma in nursing and to state registration. For the nurse who desires to specialize along either of the more advanced lines, of public health nursing, or hospital supervision and nursing education, a further period of postgraduate training is obviously desirable.

Teachers College in Columbia University has played the part of pioneer in preparing graduate nurses for hospital supervision and nursing education; and certain of the newer university schools of nursing are already offering attractive courses along the same line. The development of graduate courses in public health nursing has made even more notable progress. The first organized course of this type was offered in Boston in 1906, and by 1920 there were 20 such courses in operation, under the auspices of universities, public health nursing associations or schools of social work.

The activities of 16 of these schools of public health nursing have been studied in the course of our investigation, and the results achieved in this new field are in general deserving of high praise. The course is apparently in process of standardization at a length of about 8 months: 4 devoted to theoretical instruction in public health, public health nursing, educational psychology, and social problems; and 4 to supervised field work with a public health nursing organization. The courses at present offered are in many instances tentative and lacking in assured financial status. With the development of the university school of nursing (to be discussed in succeeding paragraphs), they may be expected to fall within its sphere of influence and to develop an increasing stability and usefulness.

Conclusion. Superintendents, supervisors, instructors, and public health nurses should in all cases receive special additional training beyond the basic nursing course.

The University School of Nursing

For advanced training the development of the University School of Nursing has been perhaps the most notable feature in the progress of nursing education during the past ten years. As long ago as 1899 Teachers College in Columbia University admitted properly qualified nurses to its junior class, thus giving 2 years of college credit for the 3 years of nursing training. Since 1916, no less than 13 different colleges and universities have provided combined courses, through which students may acquire both a nurse's training and a college degree.

The combined course in such a school, for example, involves 2 years of ordinary college work including, besides work of a liberal nature, certain of the fundamental sciences basic in nursing education. Then follow 2 years of intensive training in the hospital and, finally, a 5th year of postgraduate education in one of the higher specialties of nursing, public health, institutional supervision or nursing education. At the close of training the student receives a diploma in nursing and the bachelor's degree in nursing or in science.

This type of school of nursing should, in the judgment of the Committee, be a separate and independent department of the university, cognate in rank and organization with the school of medicine, or the school of law. It should have direct responsibility for all instruction given during the years of hospital training and the postgraduate nursing year.

A definite affiliation with one or more hospitals must in any case be established, along the line of the agreements now in force between medical schools and hospitals. The school supplies student nursing service and assumes a definite responsibility for a larger or smaller share of ward supervision and perhaps of graduate service. The hospital, on the other hand, provides maintenance for the nursing staff and conforms to the standards held by the university to be essential for the realization of its educational ideals. A university hospital will of course offer the most promising field for a university school of nursing; but in default of such an institution there seems no reason why a university school should not establish satisfactory working agreements with various adjacent hospitals, provided only that the maintenance of adequate standards in the practice field remains in its own hands.

If its present practical functions be clearly understood the university school of nursing possesses unique advantages in respect to both of the essentials for success in nursing education, to which reference has been made in a preceding paragraph. It possesses the power of independent educational leadership and is grounded on the solid foundations of educational ideals, to a degree which a training school committee, ultimately responsible to a board of hospital trustees, can seldom hope to realize; and it is likely to obtain financial resources to a more nearly adequate extent. Furthermore, through its university contacts the University School of Nursing has unique opportunities to attract students of the type so greatly needed for the fulfilment of the higher tasks in the nursing of the future.

It should be made quite clear that the Committee does not recommend that nursing schools in general should work toward the establishment of courses of a character that a university would accept for a degree. We realize that the numerical proportion of the nursing profession to be contributed by the university school will perhaps always be a relatively small one. Yet we believe that the importance of this portion of the educational structure would be difficult to overestimate. The value that we see at present in the university schools is that they will furnish a body of leaders who have the fundamental training essential in administrators, teachers, and the like. One of the greatest, if not the greatest, of the reasons for the imperfections in the present training of private duty nurses is that great numbers of schools have developed without any coincident development of adequate numbers of persons properly trained to guide the pupils during their course. Unless well taught they cannot be well trained. The university school of nursing should be the keystone of the entire arch. It will not only train leaders and develop and standardize procedures for all other schools. It will, by its permeating influence, give inspiration and balance to the movement as a whole and gradually but steadily improve the efficiency of every institution for the training of nurses of whatever type. We would therefore urge:

Conclusion. That the development and strengthening of University Schools of Nursing of a high grade for the training of leaders is of fundamental importance in the furtherance of nursing education.

Even though Josephine Goldmark pointed out many of the weaknesses that existed in the education of nurses and recommended some changes, there was no easy way to implement the recommendations contained in the report. In an overall effort to increase the quality of nursing schools, the obvious first step was to establish some sort of grading system. To do this, and to gather information for such a project, the American Nurses' Association organized a Committee on the Grading of Nursing Schools. The committee published several reports, the final one in 1934, and attempted to set minimum standards. As these standards began to be enforced many of the weaker nursing schools closed their doors.

4.

Nursing Education in the 1930's: Certain Conditions Which Should Not Be Tolerated in Schools of Nursing

Certain conditions which should not be tolerated in schools of nursing are listed below. The Grading Committee calls the attention of its national parent organizations to them. The Committee suggests that through these organizations pressure be brought to bear to close every school of nursing in which any one of these conditions *continues* to be found. The Committee believes that it is not possible to conduct such schools as educational institutions; and that such schools cannot prepare their graduates to be safely trusted with the serious responsibilities involved in the nursing care of sick people.

Not on hospital register of American Medical Association. The Committee disapproves of any hospital conducting a school of nursing unless that hospital is listed on the Hospital Register of the American Medical Association. Most reputable hospitals in this country appear on that list.

Not approved by the American College of Surgeons. The Committee disapproves of any hospital conducting a school of nursing unless that hospital is on the approved list of the American College of Surgeons. The quality of nursing education is in large measure determined by the quality of the medical and administrative staffs of the hospital which conducts the school. Failure of the hospital to receive the approval of the American College of Surgeons means either that the hospital has too few patients to be admitted to the approved lists or that the hospital has failed to recognize the importance of sound administration and of adequate professional background for the hospital and medical staff. Where these matters have not been adequately cared for, it is clear that the hospital is not yet ready to undertake the additional responsibilities of conducting an educational institution.

Not accredited by State Board of Nurse Examiners. No hospital should be allowed to conduct a school of nursing unless that school is accredited by the appropriate state agency, such as the state board of nurse examiners, and unless all the holders of the school diploma are eligible to take the state examinations for registered nurse. The practice of certain hospitals whereby they continue to conduct so-called "schools of nursing" although their gradu-

From Committee on the Grading of Nursing Schools, *Nursing Schools Today and Tomorrow.* New York: Committee on the Grading of Nursing Schools, 1934, pp. 197–213. (Extract).

ates are not eligible for the R.N. and cannot legally practice as registered nurses is dangerous and unethical. The terms "school of nursing," "training school for nurses," or similar designations which imply that the training offered prepares the graduate for admission to the nursing profession should be reserved solely for such schools as are officially approved by the state boards of nurse examiners.

Less than fifty patients. It is the opinion of the Committee that adequate clinical experience is essential for the proper education of nurses, just as it is essential for the proper education of physicians. There are many small hospitals which would be benefited by securing the services of interns; but the American Medical Association does not consider the needs of the hospital as sufficient justification for approving such institutions as training centers for interns. Similarly, the Grading Committee believes that the education of student nurses must not be sacrificed to the needs of the hospital, great as those needs may be. It is therefore the opinion of the Grading Committee that no hospital with a daily average of less than 50 patients should be permitted to conduct a school of nursing; since any hospital so small would obviously be unable to provide adequate clinical material.

The Committee has evidence to indicate that in hospitals with 50 patients or less, the cost of conducting a reasonably good school is greater than the cost of furnishing nursing service with graduates. It, therefore, does not believe that this requirement of 50 patients would work any financial hardship to the hospitals concerned. It believes that the requirement is essential for safeguarding the welfare of patients everywhere. In any state where there are no good schools conducted by hospitals with a daily average of at least 50 patients, the Committee suggests that a level of 35 patients might be taken as a first step in the process of elimination.

No training school committee. The need for some controlling board which shall have, as its chief responsibility, conduct, not of the hospital nursing service but of the school of nursing, has been demonstrated. The school should not be considered merely one of the numerous departments of the hospital. It is a project in the field of professional education and as such it demands special and continuing consideration. The Grading Committee, therefore, recommends that every school of nursing shall have a training school committee or other directing board, which shall be responsible for determining the educational policies under which the school is controlled. Such a committee, while distinct from the board of trustees of the hospital, should include in its membership some members who are members of the board, as well as some who are not.

Less than four R.N.'s. No matter how small the hospital and the school, safety for patients demands that there be at least four graduate registered nurses on the nursing and school staff. These essential four are the director of the nursing service, the day supervisor or operating room supervisor, the night supervisor, and the instructor. No school can be a good school unless it has more than these four nurses, but any school with less than these four essential nursing officers should be closed. It cannot possibly give adequate nursing care to patients or adequate training to students.

Ratio of R.N.'s to students less than 1 to 6. The larger the number of students admitted to a school, the larger the number of graduate nurses there should be. Otherwise the students will suffer from lack of adequate teaching; and the patients will suffer from unskilled and unsupervised care. Where schools conducted by large hospitals are graduating incompetent and unprofessional nurses, the reason is often to be found in the low ratio of graduate nurses to students. No hospital, whether large or small, should be permitted to conduct a school of nursing unless it employs at least one graduate nurse (including nurses on floor duty) for every six regular or affiliating students in the school. The ratio of graduates to students in any good school should be much more than this, but unless the hospital is able to provide at least one R.N. to every six students, it should not operate a school at all.

Too few hours of bedside care by nurses per patient day. No nursing school should be conducted where the care of adult bed patients (acute medical and surgical) in wards used for the training of student nurses, does not include at least an average of three hours of bedside nursing per patient, by students and graduates, in a twenty-four hour day.

In specifying this minimum ratio of nurses' time per patient, there is taken into consideration the wide variation in the needs of patients on acute medical and surgical hospital services, and the difference in hospital practices in assignment of services for patients to subsidiary workers in the wards. Without such minimum amount of nurses' care, patients lack adequate attention; and good teaching of student nurses can not be carried on.

Faculty not high school graduates. The Committee recognizes that among the older women now on the faculties of schools of nursing there are many who are excellent nurses but who have never completed full high school courses. For these women failure to possess the diploma does not necessarily imply either lack of mental ability or lack of professional interest. Among the younger nurses, however, the reverse is true. As is indicated in the recommendation which follows, the Committee believes that no student should be admitted to a school of nursing unless she possesses a high school diploma or its equivalent. The same rule should apply to all graduate nurses on the faculty who were themselves students during those recent years, in which high school education has been readily available to every capable girl.

Except for those nurses who were graduated from training school more than ten years ago, every nurse appointed to a position above the rank of general staff (or floor duty) nurse should be at least a high school graduate. Any hospital which, in the future, makes appointments which do not meet this requirement should not conduct a school of nursing. With the exception of the instructor, this ruling would not, of course, apply to nurses who are already in the employ of the hospital or of the school, but it should apply without exception to all nurses graduated from training school within the past ten years who apply for new appointments in the future.

No instructor. No hospital should conduct a school of nursing unless it provides as a member of the school faculty at least one instructor whose chief responsibility is not for administering the nursing service of the hospital, but is rather for teaching student nurses. Where the entire teaching load has to be carried by women who are also responsible for administering the nursing service of the hospital, the educational aspects of nursing are inevitably lost sight of, and the welfare of the student is repeatedly sacrificed to the nursing exigencies of the hospital. Under these conditions sound education is impossible. The Grading Committee believes that no school can be good unless it has more than one instructor; but it is essential that there be at least one such person on the school staff, whose primary concern is for the teaching of students, if the school is to be permitted to remain open.

Instructor not a high school graduate. High school education is now commonly accepted as the prerequisite for entrance to schools of nursing. Obviously the instructor must have at least as much education as the students she is to teach. It should be obvious to every one that she must have much more. The time should soon come when every school will adopt adequate educational requirements for all its faculty. In the meantime it is necessary not to jeopardize the welfare of the students by allowing the school to function where the instructor is not at least a high school graduate.

Supervisors and head nurses not R.N.'s. The Grading Committee recommends that no school shall place the direction of student nurses in the hands of other students, attendants, or practical nurses. Every nursing supervisor and every head nurse should be a graduate registered nurse. Especially does the Committee disapprove of the practice of assigning students to positions as head nurses. The head nurse has responsibility for administering the nursing service of the ward, for supervising the nursing care which patients receive, and for teaching and supervising students during their practice periods on the floors of the hospital. These responsibilities are heavy. The Committee believes that it is dangerous to the safety of the patient and deleterious to the education of the student to place this responsibility in student hands.

Students who have not completed high school. No school of nursing should

accept students who have not successfully completed a full high school education or its equivalent. While this requirement might have worked hardship on some schools a few years ago, there is ample evidence to indicate that at the present time any school which is good enough to be trusted with the education of student nurses can readily secure an adequate number of students who have met this educational requirement. Entrance requirements for good schools will demand more than mere graduation from high school, but nothing less than graduation or its equivalent should be allowed in any school. There is no shortage of high school graduates. There is no longer any reason to accept as candidates for entrance to the nursing profession young women who have not at least this minimum educational background.

No health examination on entrance. In view of the serious tuberculosis problem among nurses, annual health examinations for all student nurses, including thorough chest examinations, would seem to be essential. Certainly no school should be allowed to operate which does not give at least one such examination, under the control of its own school physicians, during the first four months the student is in the school.

School does not have at least four months' preliminary period. In order to assure safety of patients as well as protection for the student herself, the Grading Committee recommends that no hospital shall conduct a school of nursing unless it provides at least four months of preliminary instruction at the beginning of the student's training, during which time the student shall not be responsible for the care of patients. While students may assist on the wards for short periods during this time, no student should be on regular nursing duty or carry any nursing responsibilities until the four months of preliminary preparation have been completed. Assignment of students to regular nursing service before they have received this essential preparation would be sufficient reason for the state board of nurse examiners to withdraw the school from the accredited list.

Students work too many hours in each twenty-four. The Grading Committee recommends that no school shall be conducted unless it limits the regular working day or the working night of the student nurse to not more than eight hours in every twenty-four. Where students are on duty for more than eight hours in every twenty-four, they do not have enough time to do the necessary studying, and they are usually too tired to assimilate class instruction. The Committee believes that the eight-hour limit for day duty should be enforced at once. In those parts of the country where night duty is commonly conducted on a basis of more than eight hours, the Committee believes that a reasonable time limit should be set (not to exceed twelve months) in which schools can reorganize their service on the eight-hour

basis for night duty as well as for day duty. After the time limit is over, no school should be continued unless it has adopted the eight-hour maximum for night duty as well as for day duty.

Students work too many hours per week. The Committee believes that the 6-day, 48-hour working week is an inevitable and desirable maximum for graduate nurses and student nurses alike. It recommends that this standard be put into effect, and that in the meantime, no student nurses shall be assigned on active nursing service for more than 54 hours of day duty or more than 56 hours of night duty in any one week. As suggested in the preceding paragraph, reasonable time should be allowed to reorganize the weekly hours of night duty so as to bring them within the 56-hour limit, but not more than twelve months should elapse before every school has reduced its working week at least to the very moderate requirements of 54 and 56 hours recommended above.

Patients charged for student specialing. The Grading Committee condemns the practice of assigning student nurses to duty as "special" nurses in the home or in the hospital and charging the patient for such special services. Such practice not only leads to the exploitation of the student, but it interrupts her educational program. Assignments to special duty may occasionally be educationally sound, but the Committee has evidence to indicate that where student specialing is a source of financial profit there is constant temptation to assign students to such duty with little or no regard for its educational value. The Committee is convinced that this custom of charging patients for student specialing is educationally unjustifiable.

Student records not kept. Every school should keep a record for every student from the time she enters the school until she leaves it. Records in good schools will be complete and effective tools for measuring the student's progress and recording each significant development in her education. In every school, records should show at least the amounts and types of theoretical instruction and clinical experience which she has received during her training and the quality of work she has done. Until a record system covering these points is adopted, the state board of nurse examiners would be justified in withholding recognition from the school.

Diploma granted to students not eligible to state board examinations. It is the opinion of the Committee that no school should admit students who cannot become eligible, or grant its diploma to any student who is not eligible, to take examinations for registered nurse in the state where the school is located. Moreover, the signed diploma of the school should not be granted until such time as the student has actually completed her training and until she is eligible to take the state board examinations.

Not every student receives training as required by state. It is the opinion of the Grading Committee that the requirements for admission to the examinations for R.N. in most states are too low. There is therefore no good reason for being lenient with schools which fail to provide their students with even the very moderate preparation which has been prescribed by their state boards. In some states the requirements are so low that the very law which is intended as a protection to the public becomes in itself a danger, for the R.N. in such states does not assure the public that its holder is a well-qualified nurse. The R.N. is cheapened and the public is worse than unprotected.

After the Second World War, nursing education again underwent intensive study. The investigation now shifted from the problem of upgrading hospital training schools (since most schools below minimal standards were no longer in operation) to an examination of the educational qualifications for nurses. Was it enough for a nurse to have completed a basic nursing course in a recognized school of nursing? Nurses who had previously concentrated on the hospital training schools now began to examine more critically the possibilities of collegiate schools. Assisting in this was the appearance of the Association of Collegiate Schools of Nursing which was organized in 1935.

Hospital schools also found that with the proliferation of career choices for women, nursing often came off second best. More and more girls were going to college, and fewer and fewer girls were willing to enter hospital schools. It was in part the reluctance of the student to work the long hours in hospital schools that forced a raising of the standards in these schools. Colleges placed more emphasis on the collegiate aspect of their nursing programs, with the result that degree-only programs rose from 54 in 1949 to 109 in 1954 and to 177 in 1964. One of the chief forces which brought about the increase in the number of collegiate schools was a study by Margaret Bridgman.

5.
Collegiate Education for Nursing

by Margaret Bridgman

Inadequacies in the preparation of many nurses for their responsibilities are even more critical than the numerical shortages. Personnel for important functions lack both the foundation and the specialized training requisite for competence. Among nurses giving psychiatric care, including those in a super-visory capacity, 24 percent have had no preparation in their basic programs; 80 per cent have had no education in psychiatric nursing beyond the basic course. Only 34 percent of public health nurses have had preparation in an approved program of study for public health nursing. There are now approximately 70,000 administrators, teachers, supervisors, and head nurses in hospitals and schools of nursing; and it has been estimated that about half of them have had no special training for their highly specialized functions. In every phase of nursing service there is an urgent demand for more and better teachers, more efficient administrators, and more supervisors, head nurses, and clinical specialists properly equipped for their work.

The fact that more than one-fifth of all registered nurses are employed in administrative, supervisory, and teaching positions is significant evidence of the need for appropriate preparation for these functions. This proportion seems excessive until one considers that these nurses administer and supervise the services of 270,000 other nursing personnel and the care of 17,000,000 patients in hospitals, as well as nursing services to the public in public health agencies and industry. The general consensus is that the hospital diploma course is inadequate for such a purpose, but the small enrollment of students in true collegiate programs in nursing can hardly begin to meet the demand in these areas alone. There will be a still greater shortage in the fields of psychiatric and public health nursing for which also a broad foundation, particularly in the social sciences and their application in patient care, is increasingly recognized as a necessity.

The importance of providing nursing education on the college level to prepare sufficient potential candidates for such specialized functions has been repeatedly emphasized. Three recent studies of the nursing situation agreed on this need: the report of the American Medical Association on nursing problems;* *Nursing for the Future,*** by Esther Lucile Brown, which resulted

* "Report of Committee on Nursing Problems," *Journal of the American Medical Association,* vol. 137, July 3, 1948, pp. 878–879.
** Published by Russell Sage Foundation, New York, 1948.

New York: Russell Sage Foundation, 1953, pp. 25–38. (Extract).

from a nationwide survey sponsored by the National Nursing Council; and the report of the Committee on the Function of Nursing, commonly referred to as the Ginzberg Report.*

The first requirement is the establishment of baccalaureate curricula of sufficient breadth and strength to develop proficiency for expert staff nursing in hospitals, public health agencies, and other services and to provide a sound base for graduate study, in general and profession-related content and in nursing as the major field of concentration. Experience and competence on the staff level are essential as a foundation for the larger responsibilities of supervision, administration, teaching, clinical specialization, and research. To provide a source of supply for advanced positions, there must be considerably more students in undergraduate programs than will be ultimately needed to fill the positions. Allowance must be made for normal attrition and there should also be an opportunity for a selective process by which students with distinctive abilities and interests would be encouraged to secure advanced preparation. Some college graduates prefer the direct care of patients to administrative and teaching functions, and their choice of work should be free from pressures. Moreover, expert clinicians with a broad educational background are urgently needed for research functions in nursing to contribute to medical research, to segregate and analyze the components of good nursing care, and to contribute the specific knowledge and skills requisite for various kinds of nursing.

The reasons that sound basic collegiate education is required for the most skilled duties of the professional nurse and for advancement are little understood by the public or by educators generally. As previously noted, the isolation of nursing education from educational institutions has prevented intercommunication between teachers and students in this area with those in others— the natural means of mutual understanding and of disseminating knowledge about the purposes, methods, and needs in an educational program and the occupation for which it prepares. Few realize the changes that have taken place within recent years in the scope and nature of nursing care.

Scientific and technological advances have revolutionized medical practice and every new development in medicine creates new responsibilities for nursing. The process of turning over more and more technical procedures to nurses began in the seventies and eighties of the past century with the introduction of antiseptic and aseptic techniques. Temperature-taking was at first delegated with caution. The giving of hypodermics soon followed. The extraordinarily rapid medical developments during and since the last war have given a strong impetus to this movement. Physicians throughout the

* *A Program for the Nursing Profession.* Macmillan Co., New York, 1948.

country testify to the fact that many procedures, some of them extremely complex, which previously belonged exclusively to medical practice, are now entrusted to nurses. The proportion of acutely ill patients in hospitals has very greatly increased because of the quick recoveries made possible by the use of new drugs and therapeutic measures, and also because of current policies in regard to early ambulation and discharge. The heavy demands upon doctors and the constant or frequent attention required in present diagnostic and therapeutic practices necessitate the transfer of many clinical procedures to nurses. For example, penicillin injections were first delegated to nurses at night because doctors were not regularly available. Then the absurdity of the belief that nurses were not capable of taking this responsibility in the day-time was recognized. In large medical centers some of these procedures are carried on by interns and resident doctors, but in the smaller hospitals they are routinely performed by nurses. All professional nurses must know how to administer such treatments.

There is a borderline area between medical and nursing practice in which there is at present disagreement among physicians which results in confusion and inconsistencies. Intravenous therapy, for instance, including such procedures as saline injections and blood transfusions, is considered by some to be exclusively medical practice. Others think it can be performed by nurses under medical direction and supervision, and still others delegate it regularly to competent nurses. In an emergency nurses have to carry out these procedures to save life, as they did in World War II, and they must be prepared to do so in an atomic disaster or in any situation where the services of a physician are not available.* Most schools of nursing therefore teach students the methods but nurses are expected to conform to medical policies that prevail where they are working.

The kind of responsibility required of nurses is indicated by the fact that even those in first-level staff positions, that is, immediately after graduation from a school of nursing, are expected to perform a long list of duties upon order of a physician or dentist but without medical supervision, subject only to medical policies as indicated above. This list includes administration of therapeutic measures in a way appropriate to the type, amount, frequency, sequence, technique, and method approved by the medical staff. Such measures include medications by mouth, subcutaneously, intradermally, intramuscularly, intravenously, rectally, topically, by inhalation; applications of heat, cold, and pressure; therapeutic baths and exercises; surgical dressings; and irrigations of body cavities. Nurses must also keep up with new nursing techniques

---

* See "Should Nurses Do Venipunctures?" *American Journal of Nursing*, vol. 51, October, 1951, pp. 603–604. (Opinions of authorities in American Medical Association and American Hospital Association.)

introduced by rapidly changing medical practice and developed in consultation with the physicians concerned.

Nursing care given to patients undergoing treatments involves complex equipment as, for example, for those in respirators or for those requiring tracheotomy or other intubation or therapy with radium or oxygen. Nurses must prevent improper or overuse of such equipment and observe the reaction of the patient during and after treatment so as to preclude shock, hemorrhage, unconsciousness, and so forth. They also administer diagnostic tests such as the Mantoux, Dick, and Schick. All these duties are in addition to those in which they contribute to the medical evaluation of the patient's condition and progress by determining, recording, and reporting temperature, pulse, respiration, blood pressure, visual acuity, hearing and color perception, as well as by noting signs and symptoms of acute complications or deviations from the usual process of convalescence.

Nurses are required to know how to prepare patients for various types of surgery, with or without specific instructions. An error in an order does not absolve them from responsibility concerning the properties of drugs and the conditions of their safe administration. Visitors to classes in nursing are frequently impressed by the number of times instructors repeat emphatically, "This is the nurse's responsibility. You are expected to know this procedure without specific directions."

The common impression that the hospital nurse is constantly under medical supervision is far from correct. A brief visit each day from the patient's physician is usual practice, and in hospitals having no resident staff this visit constitutes the only supervision of the nurse's care of the patient. Doctors rely on nurses to summon them in an emergency and also to take immediate measures, before their arrival, if a critical situation demands them. Acutely ill postsurgical patients in "recovery rooms" are frequently not seen by a physician for eight hours after the operation unless called by a nurse. Nurses carry particularly heavy responsibilities at night.

To become able professional nurses, students need a good foundation in the biological and physical sciences, in pharmacology and therapeutics, and enough knowledge of medical science so that they will thoroughly understand what they are doing. Certainly it is necessary for teaching and directing others. Mechanical skills can be learned without this foundation, but the understanding of the reasons for, and the effects of, one's work is essential for intelligent and effective performance. A great deal of supervision becomes necessary when procedures are carried on by personnel who do not have adequate knowledge or cannot be relied on for good judgment. The stimulus to assume responsibility is also lacking in learning and practicing by rote. The satisfaction a nurse derives from applying full knowledge to the solution of a patient's problem helps to keep her interest keen, aids in preventing careless mistakes, and supports her in disregarding personal fatigue.

Current studies of the interaction of the mental, emotional, and physical aspects of health and disease, and the effects of social, economic, religious, and other cultural influences emphasize the importance of ministering to the patient's total needs. The nurse has opportunities to develop a therapeutic relationship with the patient that may be a significant and even a decisive factor in his progress, if she has learned the values and methods of the sociopsychosomatic approach through effective study and guided application of sociological and psychological principles.

The ability to give "supportive care" to patients of all kinds and ages, under varied circumstances, and with infinitely varied characteristics, is increasingly recognized as a significant qualification of a professional nurse. The realization that fear creates unpredictable hazards in a surgical operation, that emotional tensions may impede or even prevent recovery, that sometimes life itself is more dependent on the will to live than upon physical conditions, and in general the recognition that a patient is a human being with a mind, a heart, and a spirit, not just a diseased body, has given added importance to the need for as much wisdom as possible in helping him meet the crisis of illness with an attitude contributing positively to recovery and continued health of mind and body.

Students who are taught to apply psychological principles to the understanding of personality differences, the characteristics of various stages of life, emotional problems, minor deviations from the normal, and finally, in psychiatric nursing, the treatment and care of seriously maladjusted people, have a basis for understanding their patients' needs. If they acquire an insight that enables them to adjust satisfactorily themselves and to exert a positive influence on others—patients, their families, and coworkers—in the complex interpersonal relationships and emotional tensions of a hospital, they can contribute largely to therapeutic conditions. They also gain a foundation for, and frequently an interest in, psychiatric nursing which make them potential candidates for specialization in that field and for positions in mental hospitals where, as already noted, there is so urgent a need for qualified personnel.

Health teaching as part of the nurse's role is gaining in importance with emergent conceptions of the responsibilities of the health services for the maintenance of health, not merely for treating disease during the acute stages. The continuity previously provided by the family physician, convalescence in the hospital, and by a nurse in accompanying the patient home has been largely lost in an age of specialists, brief hospital stays, and both economic and personnel limitations on home care. The necessity for making more adequate provisions for the patient's welfare after hospitalization is very apparent.

The increased strain upon hospital facilities focuses attention upon the urgency of developing inclusive and continuous community health programs in which the functions of the hospital are closely correlated with those of other agencies for public health and welfare. Health education; immunization to control communicable disease; early discovery of serious maladies; out-patient treatment of transient or chronic illness; mental hygiene, maternal, well-baby, and other clinics; visiting nurse services; social services—all have a part in such programs. In some communities hospitals are becoming centers for coordinated health activities, as well as establishing relationships with other agencies so that there may be greater breadth and more effective con-tinuity in the services offered the public.

The nurse has a significant function in such inclusive health programs, within the hospital, in the outpatient department, and in the public health field. Of great importance is adequate preparation, such as is being provided by integration of public health nursing in baccalaureate curricula, not only to qualify graduates for beginning positions in that area but to add competence for every type of nursing. The nurse needs to understand the social factors affecting the patient, to know community conditions and resources. She often has an opportunity to discover problems and contribute to their solution either directly or by enlisting the aid of others. Frequently she has a large share in teaching patients and their families practices and attitudes that will promote recovery, rehabilitation (sometimes with difficult adjustments to physical limitations), and continued health after their return home.

A doctor recently described the success of a nurse in creating such attitudes in a young woman badly crippled by poliomyelitis. She had received a severe shock through overhearing a thoughtless reference to herself as a "hopeless case." The nurse, however, taught her ways of overcoming her disabilities and imparted such courage and confidence to her, and wisdom to her husband, that she is now able, though confined to a wheelchair, to care for her children, to perform household tasks with specially built facilities, and to be the center of an exceptionally happy family.

In one instance known to the writer the faculty of a collegiate school of nursing, which utilizes through contractual agreement the facilities of a large hospital for the instruction and supervised practice of the students, has taken the initiative in securing the approval of the medical staff in the formulation of materials that nurses are authorized to use in the instruction of patients and their families concerning posthospital care in various diseases and conditions. These teaching outlines are more inclusive than the pamphlets given to patients themselves and have proved very valuable in saving the doctor's time and in clarifying and defining the nurse's responsibilities. Consultations with the sick person enable the nurses to adapt their guidance to his actual living conditions. Often, with the physician's direction or approval, the nurse coordinates other consultation services, such as those of a dietitian and a social worker who contribute to a complete and practicable plan for the patient's convalescence, return to full or partial activity, and maintenance of maximum health. Referrals to a public health or social agency or both may be involved, in which case the nurse and the social worker, if there is one, communicate pertinent information to those who will carry on the care and guidance.

In another hospital a group of graduate nurses became concerned about the difficulties—physical, emotional, and social—experienced by patients with a colostomy. They organized a committee including a surgeon, the department head of medical and surgical nursing, graduate staff nurses, social worker, dietitian, and others to consider the problem. The task of investigation and formulation of specific recommendations was delegated to a smaller work committee of nurses, under the chairmanship of the supervisor of surgical nursing. A careful study was made of techniques, and devices and methods were evolved that are well adapted to enable a person with this distressing disability to use effective hygienic procedures, avoid embarrassment, and lead a normal, active life. The chairman of this committee is now recognized as a valuable consultant for such patients, not only by surgeons in her own hospital but by others. Instruction begins before surgery, is continued in the hospital, and later in the home by a visiting nurse who has been fully informed of the patient's individual problems and family situation. The success of this project has given marked encouragement for the development of plans for teaching patients with other types of illness to care for themselves and manage their lives more satisfactorily.*

* See Dericks, Virginia C., and Kathryn A. Robeson, "Problems of Colostomy Patients," *Public Health Nursing,* January, 1949.

The growth of collegiate education for nurses did not halt the persistent shortage of nurses. The majority of nurses are still graduated from hospital schools. These schools, faced with continual upgrading, more rigid screening, and more costly programs, are reluctant to increase the size of their classes. Moreover, many nurses feel that it is manifestly unfair for other professions to be educated in tax-supported institutions while nurses are still, for the most part, educated in private or church-sponsored hospitals, and when they are educated in tax-supported hospitals they are given little support by the community. Because of this situation, an increasing number of nurses began to look at the community or junior colleges as training grounds for nurses. These had the advantage of being community oriented; they were tax supported, and were proliferating across the continent. Instrumental in establishing the junior college program was Mildred L. Montag. The concept of the junior college, however, has reopened many of the old controversies in nursing. Is a two year community college program equivalent to a three- or four-year hospital school? What distinctions exist between the junior college R.N., the hospital school R.N., and the collegiate R.N.?

6.

Community College Education for Nursing

by Mildred L. Montag and Lassar G. Gotkin

The Cooperative Research Project in Junior and Community College Education for Nursing had as its purpose the development and testing of a new type of program preparing young men and women for those functions commonly associated with the registered nurse. The term *bedside nurse* has also been used to describe the kind of nurse that would be prepared by this new program. This term is intended to imply certain limitations of activity that differentiate the role of this nurse from that of the nurse with broader professional preparation. It was felt that there is a function to be performed by many registered nurses (not practical nurses or aides) in giving direct care to patients, where these nurses have access to the supervision of other nurses more broadly prepared. This should not be taken to imply, however, that nurses with broad professional preparation will not give direct care to patients.

There is growing interest and effort within the nursing profession to realign education for nursing in harmony with changing functions in nursing. The need for the nurse who is able to perform the professional functions of nursing is clear. Equally clear is the need for those to carry on the technical, or semi-professional, functions, and it is in this area that great numbers of nurses are needed. Therefore, the move toward the development of both the four-year, professional type of program and the shorter, semi-professional type is consistent with the need for nurses to carry on the whole range of nursing functions. It is with the latter type of program that this project has been concerned.

Certain assumptions were basic to the development of the proposal for the project. Others were identified by the project advisory committee in its first meeting. The assumptions which underlie the whole project are:

1. The functions of nursing can and should be differentiated into three basic categories: the professional, the semi-professional or technical, the assisting.

2. The great bulk of nursing functions lie in the intermediate category, the semi-professional or technical. Therefore, the greatest number of persons should be prepared to fulfill these functions.

3. Education for nursing belongs within the organized educational framework.

4. The junior-community college, the post-high school educational institution specifically suited to semi-professional or technical education, is the logical institution for the preparation of the large group of nurses.

5. When preparation for nursing is education—rather than service-centered, the time required may be reduced.

The aims of the project, as accepted by the advisory committee in conference with the staff, were concerned primarily with the graduates of the new type of program. It was hoped that the graduates would qualify for the registered nurse's license, meet the junior-community college requirements for the associate degree, perform technical (or semi-professional) functions at the registered-nurse level, be prepared for beginning practitioner positions (with supervision and, if possible, in situations where in-service training would be available), and, on graduation, be prepared to *become* competent nurses rather than *be* fully competent.

A last anticipated outcome had to do with the program itself: This new type of program would be terminal, but qualified individual graduates would be eligible for professional education in nursing at the upper-division level.

• • •

The need for nurses has increased steadily through the years and the discrepancy between the supply of nurses and the need for nursing services has become increasingly apparent. To maintain the present ratio of nurses to population in future years will require an increase in the number of nurses proportionate to the increase in population. The present enrollment in schools of nursing gives little evidence that the need can be met without changes either in the way nurses are prepared or in the institutions involved in preparing nurses.

● ● ●

The community college is said to be the "fastest-growing collegiate enterprise in America today." Its major purpose is to meet the community's needs for essential services. It is with this institution that the Cooperative Research Project worked to develop new nursing programs. The new programs represent a change in the way nurses are prepared and a new responsibility on the part of junior-community colleges for the education of nurses.

The conclusions which appear justified on the basis of the findings of the present study are:

1. Nurses able to carry on the functions commonly associated with the registered nurse can be prepared in the new type nursing program conducted by the junior-community college. They are able to pass licensing examinations successfully, and with some experience, they are able to carry on the nursing functions as well as or better than the graduates of other types of nursing programs with the same purpose.

2. These programs attract students. The applications to the programs have consistently exceeded the number that could be admitted, and enrollments have increased and are increasing. Furthermore, certain individuals who might otherwise not have been attracted to or able to attend another type of nursing school found these programs particularly desirable and accessible.

3. Nursing programs of this type can be set up as integral curricula in junior and community colleges. From an administrative point of view, it is possible to set up a nursing program as a department or division which can operate within the organizational framework of the college. From the point of view of the curricular organization, the general education requirement can be combined practically with the vocationally oriented nursing courses. The nursing courses can be set up within the framework of the total curriculum, using the same time and credit allowances as used in other courses. From the student's point of view, becoming a nurse in the community college setting is particularly gratifying. The inclusion of general education courses, taken with students of other programs, is desirable and helpful.

4. Junior-community colleges have found it possible to finance these programs within the financial structure of the institution. No particular

study of costs has been made, but the administrators of several colleges have pointed out that while the nursing program is not the least expensive program, neither is it the most expensive. The cost of the nursing program is quite in keeping with the cost of other specialized programs. One president stated that the nursing program was less expensive, for example, than the specialized electronic technician program.

5. It is possible to utilize the facilities of hospitals and other health agencies for the learning experiences desired without payment of fees or through service by students. What cost has been incurred by the agency in the use of its facilities has been offset in part by services which result as a by-product of the student's learning experiences. The hospitals have recognized the need for the product of these nursing programs and have accepted their social obligation to provide their facilities without charge. They also recognize the intangible but very real value accrued from the added stimulation of the nursing staff.

6. Where nursing service understands and accepts the concept of a graduate nurse as a beginning practitioner at the time of graduation and not a finished product, the graduate of the junior-community college nursing program is oriented more realistically and absorbed more quickly into the nursing service.

The conclusions reached in a study are based on the data collected and evaluated. Equally important, though probably less specific, are the implications which these conclusions have. What use is made of the study and its findings is perhaps more significant than the study itself. Obviously all the possible implications cannot be seen at this time, and so no attempt has been made at all-inclusiveness. However, some of the implications of this study for nursing education generally, for junior-community college education, for nursing service, and for the nursing profession will be pointed out.

Nursing Education

Nursing education has been under scrutiny many times in its history but never more so than in the last decade. In spite of concern about where nursing programs should be and what they should do, the Cooperative Research Project in Junior and Community College Education for Nursing marked the first systematic attempt to develop a new type program in a new setting. It is true that a considerable number of junior colleges have been involved in some way in nursing programs for many years, but it is also true that the programs developed in junior-community colleges in the project are completely new and not a continuation or even a revision of those programs previously carried on in this type of institution. Neither are they shortened versions of the traditional three-year hospital program. It would be a great mistake if nursing educators and hospital administrators saw this new program only as a shortened program and consequently believed that their own nursing programs could easily be converted to two-year programs. It is unfortunate that more emphasis has been given to the shorter length of the program than to its changed philosophy.

One of the strongest implications of these five years of experimentation is the need for a clear statement of the objectives of each type of nursing program. The statement of objectives is dependent on a clear picture of the product to be produced by the educational program and of the functions this product should perform. We can no longer have programs differing in length, content, and method and yet claiming to be preparing professional practitioners of the same competency. Until and unless the objectives of the several programs can be differentiated, there can be little argument for the continuation of multiple programs. There can be little justification for a program in nursing which requires four years for its completion unless that program prepares a practitioner who is different in competence from the graduate of the junior college program. There is little evidence to support the belief that in the majority, at least, of the present four-year programs this is the case.

The question of what the four-year or baccalaureate degree program should be is not easily answered. There are suggestions made that the baccalaureate degree program has wider cultural and general education advantages and that the time spent is justifiable. Others suggest that the graduate of the baccalaureate degree program becomes the nurse-manager and therefore believe that the program should include courses in management. To accept either of these conclusions is to misunderstand the question or to underestimate its seriousness. Still another proposal is made which is commonly referred to as the "ladder concept." This plan would make it possible for students to enter programs designed to permit the completion of one year with employment possible thereafter as practical nurses; the completion of two years permitting licensure as a registered nurse; an additional two years providing for courses in management and teaching. There is in this plan considerable confusion about the objectives and methodology of technical and professional education. That there is a difference in nature, scope and purpose between these two types of education is well known. It is difficult to understand why nurse educators and others believe the two can appropriately be carried on within a single program. If curricula are built upon objectives and content and teaching methods are selected accordingly, then the ladder concept of curricular development is indefensible. The decision whether there is a place for the professional practitioner in nursing must be made, and programs set up to prepare those who wish to function at that level. The recent study by Lambertsen* should be extremely useful in clarifying the role of the professional practitioner and in planning an educational program for that role.

Almost all criticisms of the pilot programs have been concerned with time. It has been said that the program is not long enough, that not enough time is spent in the clinical situation, and that nursing cannot be learned in so short a time. Much more rare, almost to the point of nonexistence, have been comments about the quality of the content, the instruction, and the learning experiences. It has been demonstrated in the pilot programs that less learning time is needed when the learning experiences are carefully selected and organized and when the teacher and student can concentrate on teaching and learning. It therefore seems obvious that the reliance on time-spent units as the sole criterion for the quality of a course or set of experiences is wholly unjustifiable. Noteworthy progress away from such arbitrary time limits has been made by the American Nurses' Association Special Committee on State Boards of Nursing in their recommendations for standards.** It now remains for the state boards of nursing to revise their standards accordingly.

However, great harm can be done to nursing programs and to nursing if the notion gains currency that the simple elimination of the third year is equivalent to what has been done in the pilot programs. Because the junior college program has been attractive to students for a variety of reasons, it cannot be assumed that hospital nursing programs can attract students by the simple expedient of shortening the program. The success of the junior college programs and that of the one hospital included in the Cooperative Research Project is by no means a directive for hospitals either to shorten existing programs or to set up new two-year programs. When the nursing program at Monmouth Memorial Hospital is carefully analyzed, it will be seen to resemble the college programs very closely. Therefore, unless a hospital wishes to reorganize its nursing education program completely and, in essence, establish an independent school of nursing, it should not consider a two-year program at all.

Whether a hospital should carry on a nursing education program at all still remains to be answered. Can the hospital justify the expenditures necessary for a good nursing program? Is this a legitimate use for money the hospital receives? It was an assumption basic to this project that education for

* Eleanor C. Lambertsen, "Professional Education for Leadership in the Practice of Nursing." Unpublished doctoral project, Teachers College, Columbia University, 1957.
** A.N.A. Special Committee on State Boards of Nursing, "Progress Report of the Subcommittee on the Preparation of Educational Standards to be Used as a Guide by State Boards." Mimeographed, May 1956.

nursing is the legitimate obligation of educational institutions and experiences since have done nothing to lessen the acceptability of this assumption.

An important question arising from the pilot programs has been that of the interneship. Several junior-community colleges have indicated their intention of including a year's internship so that the over-all time required would remain three years. This has been suggested for two basic reasons— first, to meet the state board of nursing requirement of a three-year period, and, second, to avoid the criticism and opposition of nurses and nursing groups.

Hospital administrators have expressed considerable interest in the interneship. This is understandable since an internship would assure them of the services of a given number of nurses for a year, and then an easy replacement with succeeding groups of internes. Findings of this study show that students in the practicum were functioning as graduate nurses, and they were so considered in the evaluation. That the internship is a period ripe for exploitation is all too evident.

Nurses who advocate an internship may be doing so because of the nature of their own educational program. When time spent in the various services within a hospital is the only matter of concern in setting up or in evaluating a nursing program, it is scarcely surprising that the graduates of such programs stress time. Unfortunately, nursing programs have been more controlled by the time element than have any other educational programs. Perhaps as nursing programs come increasingly under the direction of educational institutions, the question of time will take its proper place.

• • •

Nursing Service

This project was not primarily concerned with nursing service, except as it was concerned with the preparation of personnel able to carry out the functions of the registered nurse. In the course of the project, as various hospitals were used to provide laboratory experiences for students and, more particularly, during the evaluation study of the graduates, many observations were made of nursing services. One of the most obvious observations was the vast amount of nursing care given by other than registered nurses. It was common to find nursing students carrying out functions comparable to those of practical nurses and aides, with registered nurses carrying on only managerial tasks. It is disturbing to find graduates of all kinds of nursing programs identifying the time they either were head nurses or relieved the head nurse as the time they assumed full nursing responsibility. It is apparently the common belief that direct care of patients lies outside the scope of the functions of the registered nurse. That the nursing service has promoted this idea, or at least condoned it, seems obvious. The purpose of the project was to prepare the bedside nurse, for it was felt that the need for this kind of nurse was great. The graduates expressed pleasure in giving direct care to patients and concern when they were not permitted to do so because auxiliary personnel were so assigned.

Nursing service must answer the question of who shall give direct nursing care to patients. If all nursing care is to be given by auxiliary nursing personnel, are they not, in effect, nurses? Is there not a place at the bedside for the highly skilled technician and for the professional nurse as well? A convincing argument for the nurse's doing nursing is made by Lambertsen on the basis of several years of study and experience with the nursing team.* It is not enough to place the blame for the present situation on the so-called shortage of nurses. It is a problem much less easily solved than that. It requires a re-evaluation of what constitutes nursing care, and by whom it should be given. At the conclusion of this project, there is no change in the belief that there is a need for the registered nurse at the bedside. There is strengthened belief that the nurse must be permitted to do nursing and to do it well if she is to receive satisfaction from the job of nursing and to wish to continue in it. Those responsible for nursing service will have to find ways and means of organization that will permit nurses to nurse.

There has been a great deal of discussion in recent years about in-service education in hospital nursing service. Public health nursing agencies have long since assumed the continued education of their personnel as one of their responsibilities. Hospital nursing services have not felt this need particularly because so many hospitals have schools of nursing which prepare their own personnel. In fact, in the past, most hospital schools have prepared nurses specifically for their own institutions and not for nursing generally. It was common practice for graduates to spend all, or almost all, of their professional life employed by the hospital in which they were trained. The reduction in the number of schools of nursing, the increase in the number of hospitals, and the greater mobility of nurses have changed this picture considerably. Now less than one-fifth of all hospitals have schools of nursing, and personnel must be secured from other institutions. Moreover, the medical treatment of patients has changed drastically and continues to change at an unprecedented rate. With these changes, nursing care must also change. A nurse specifically prepared today may find herself ill equipped tomorrow. As the nursing service is organized increasingly as specialized services, the difference between units within the same institution is often as great as or greater than that between institutions. The nurse will need orientation to

* Lambertsen, *op. cit.*

and continued education in the service in which she is working. Because of the great degree of specialization, nursing programs must increasingly be concerned with basic nursing care, with specialization coming after graduation as a result of in-service or continuing training. The need for continuing education is not a matter of choice, it is a matter of necessity.

There seems to have been a verbal or intellectual acceptance of in-service education or continuing education by nursing service administrators. It is unfortunate that there has not been accompanying understanding, for in too many institutions in-service education is only a word. Some institutions have a plan on paper, but it has not been implemented nor is there a real intention of doing so. In some institutions the concept of in-service education is a series of lectures. In others there is admittedly no plan at all. In all three types of situations, shortage of personnel and shortage of time are given as justification for doing so little in this area. The strongest implication of this study for the nursing service seems to be the need for a vigorous, dynamic, farsighted and imaginative plan of in-service education.

● ● ●

The Nursing Profession

The responsibility of a profession for the service it renders to society through its members is a well-accepted principle. Thus a profession is responsible for the education of its members. The nursing profession may well find implications for the practice of nursing from the results of the Cooperative Research Project.

Perhaps the first and most obvious inference to be made is the need for study of what the role and functions of the nurse should be. The seeming reluctance of registered nurses to give direct care to patients, and the preference for service and institutional managerial functions, should cause concern in the profession. To what extent will nurses take on functions the physicians discards? To what extent will nurses be drawn into management beyond that of the nursing of her patient? Will nurses of the future nurse, or, as some studies indicate, merely see that nursing gets done—by some other group? The nursing profession cannot afford simply to let changes come about or even be forced on it. It will have to look into the future and make plans to bring about the changes it considers best.

The statments of functions which have been developed by the various sections of the American Nurses Association are important statements. They should be more than words; they should be major agreements which govern the practice of nursing. At the beginning of the Cooperative Research Project the junior college presidents asked for just such statements so that their nursing programs could be planned to prepare nurses to perform those functions ascribed to the general staff nurse. At that time no such statements were available. It is questionable even now whether these agreements as to functions are well known to the practicing nurse or are in any way affecting what the nurse does or does not do.

One of the chief merits of the statements of functions is that in each category the nurses actually engaged in that branch of nursing were responsible for developing the statement. This is as it should be, for if the profession is to be self-controlled it must have the participation of the practitioner in decisions relating to the practice of nursing within the framework of the rightful province of other professions.

Nursing educators have probably not been as cognizant of these statements of functions as they should be. Curricular development in the schools of nursing is dependent on such decisions as the practitioner makes, for it is for the practice of nursing that the students are being prepared. Thus the statements of functions become, or should become, curricular guides.

The attraction of persons to a profession and the admission of those eligible is another responsibility of a profession. From the findings in this project, it seems obvious that changes in recruitment policies and procedures are in order. There has been an apparent reluctance, or at least too little emphasis, on the part of the profession to encourage either the development of nursing programs in colleges or the direction of attention toward such programs in recruitment activities. The evidence supporting collegiate programs seems clear. The slowness of the development of college-centered programs in nursing has not been equalled by any other profession.

The profession must recognize too the differences between professional and semi-professional or technical functions and between professional and technical education. There are specific ways in which a professional person performs the functions ascribed to that profession. To be able to function in this way is one of the outcomes of professional education. It does not just happen; it requires a deliberately planned training. Nurses are frequently disturbed by any implication that all nursing functions are not professional in nature and that all nurses are not professional people. Simply to label a function professional or to name a person professional, either by law or custom, does not make them so. The recognition that there are differentiated functions within the occupation of nursing is a first step. It follows naturally that preparation for these different categories of functions must be differentiated. A natural consequence of these two is that in the practice of nursing, provision must be made for these nurses to work together. That there can be careers in either professional or semi-professional nursing should be clear.

The nursing profession finds itself in a challenging position. What it does within the next few years may determine its entire future. Whether it will become a profession or whether it will abrogate its place and position to another group is within its power to determine. It is an exciting time to be in nursing. It is a discouraging time to be in nursing. Changes are needed so badly and they seem so obvious and so possible. Yet changes seem to be discouraged—or at least not encouraged—by so many in the field of nursing. The decision as to how the profession will move is in the hands of the nurses themselves.

> Most nurses are still trained by the hospital diploma schools and the hospitals will undoubtedly continue to play an important if not major role in the training of nurses.

7.

A Reaffirmation of Belief in the Diploma School of Nursing

by Ruth Sleeper

The women and men who are being graduated from diploma programs constitute the very heart of nursing in the hospitals of this country. Often their number determines whether hospital beds are available or closed to the public. To the doctor, our graduates represent the core of the patient care team. Without question they staff the services on which nursing students from all types of educational programs receive their clinical experience.

Why, if all of this is true, does anyone question the continuance of the diploma program? If we do not question its continuance, why do we not have ready firm, convincing answers when we are asked questions about it? What has happened to our faith in our products, in our future, in ourselves? Why do our convictions desert us whenever a new form of education for nurses is introduced? Why do we look so eagerly at the new, and so disparagingly at our own programs?

What are we seeking—prestige, or sound products; status in educational circles, or respect for a necessary job well done; change for change's sake, or change in our own programs which will provide graduate nurses who are better able to fill the health needs today, in 1960, or in 1980? Why has

Reprinted, with permission, from *Nursing Outlook, VI*, 1958, 616–618.

it taken us five years to make clear to all concerned our belief in our program?

Are we thinking soundly, or has someone with an air of strong conviction said to us recently, "Give up the diploma program; change to university or junior college?" Or, perhaps someone has said, "Remember, the National League for Nursing publication, *Nurses for a Growing Nation,* says that degree graduates must increase from 15 percent to 33 percent, and diploma graduates decrease from 85 percent to 67 percent."

Let us not be misled. We believe in university programs; we believe in junior college programs. We also know that these figures, as quoted, can be misleading. This publication discusses future needs which will require that annual admissions to basic nursing schools rise from the current level of 45,000 to about 70,000. Figure it out for yourselves; 85 percent of 45,000 admissions falls short of 67 percent of 70,000 admissions by over 8000 students. What *Nurses for a Growing Nation* is really saying is that annual admissions to diploma schools must be stepped up by over 8000.

Of course, these misleading statements are often made by those who are not directly responsible for staffing hospital wards, by persons who are not responsible for conducting a diploma school. In short, many of those who make these statements are least familiar with the intimate details of supply and demand for nurses. My own reaction then is one of considerable emotion. On what basis do we make our decisions? This is no small matter. It is a question of upsetting an educational system which has produced nurses for our country for 83 years. This system is assured at least reasonable support, and often generous moral and financial support. It is also a question of giving up a familiar, and a much needed, system without adequate provision to replace it. In fact, no one really knows how rapidly or slowly other schools could be developed to replace the hospital-conducted school, nor does anyone know what proportion of the new product would consent to carry the direct nursing care which is provided now by the diploma school graduates.

We, who live close to sick people in hospitals, close to the various fields of science which serve these people, and close to the thousands of nurses who have been graduated from diploma programs will surely not wish to make hurried, unwise decisions. We must take time to look at our beliefs, our methods, our future plans.

What is wrong with the diploma program? Many reasons are given. Some say, "It is old style." But it is not necessarily senescent unless we make it so. "It is supported by a service agency," we are told. But so, in part, though usually in a different way and to a lesser degree, are medicine, physical therapy, pharmacy, and several other disciplines. "Our situation," say diploma school faculty, "is different in that other forms of nursing education initiate in a university or college, which is the accepted pattern for *all* education."

But is it wrong to have a variety of patterns? It is a single-purpose school, we know, and lacks breadth of contacts for living and for education which the multipurpose school in the university can provide, but it attracts many young women and men who could not, or would not, go to college whatever the time, expense, or other requirements might be.

The diploma program is criticized because it differs financially, since the student receives certain perquisites for which students in college pay. But if the need is for more nurses, and more candidates for nursing can afford this plan of education, shall we deny them and lose this supply for our communities?

More practice time is sometimes demanded of the students in hospital schools than is consistent with good education, they tell us. But should we condemn an entire system because one aspect is wrong, or because some of the schools fail to meet their obligations to their students? Or, should we try to make the situation right?

Frankly, if each aspect of the hospital diploma program is analyzed, wrong really occurs not because the hospital runs the school, but because the school itself fails to provide a sound educational program. This is just as true when the school under scrutiny is conducted by a university or a junior college. Remember, I am for all three types.

I have often tried to determine why we have so much confusion in our educational system in nursing. We say that the public is confused. Then, I wonder who clarifies the situations for them? We say that the hospital administrator does not understand. Then, I ask myself who clarifies our belief for him back home in his own institution? We say that the nurses misunderstand, yet who are these nurses but ourselves? What are we going to do about it all?

The diploma program was the pioneer. To be sure, Miss Nightingale's original plan was changed as schools opened hurriedly in the early years. Much in her philosophy and purpose was lost or modified. Nevertheless, much in those early schools will still stand up against contemporary criteria of the times. A little of the philosophy and purpose illustrated by those early schools might even stand firmly if they were measured by the criteria of 1958.

Trying to judge the programs of 25, 10, or even 5 years ago by today's criteria is a little like studying a near object under a field glass. The object as a whole cannot be seen, but its flaws stand out so starkly as to make the whole seem imperfect. This is an exaggerated picture rather than a valid one. On the other hand, it does not pay to turn the field glass wrong end to, as the child enjoys doing. In this distorted view the whole is seen clearly, but at such a distance that no true judgment can be made. The whole looks perfect. This might be called the sentimental view, and not a valid one either.

When nursing education was introduced in the hospital school, it made a contribution to the health needs of the people as judged by contemporary criteria. Then came the university school, at first of the affiliation type. These early university schools offered few differences other than the opportunity provided for broader science teaching, a taste of liberal arts study, and some exposure to college life. Then followed the more soundly organized 5- and 4-year programs.

Unfortunately, the hospital schools looked at these newcomers in the universities as examples with more prestige. It was believed that the university school graduate had greater status. Too often the diploma school, eager to have the best for its students, strove to add everything, or imitate too many of the innovations without regard for its differing objectives. The public, and the candidates for nursing, and the hospital family as a whole wanted to know what was the difference between the diploma and the degree program.

There is, I believe, a difference which is of great importance. Certainly there should be a difference, for one student invests more in time, academic effort, and money than the other. Surely the university program should be worth this added investment. Yet this fact should neither belittle the product nor reduce the value of the investment made in the diploma school.

One difference should lie, first of all, in the purpose of the two programs (diploma and degree) as derived from the philosophies of the schools. We, in the diploma program are agreed, I believe, that we should prepare the bedside nurse. So far as I know this has always been true. The university school, with its broad opportunities, should prepare for more rapid progress to positions of leadership. Existing in a democracy, our diploma schools will produce leaders also, and these young women and men will seek and enjoy opportunities for college study and, if desired, advanced specialization. However, direct care of patients should continue to be the basic purpose of the diploma school.

To find our objectives, then, we would naturally look first at the needs of patients. As we in diploma schools are also interested in, and aware of the value of, sound teaching methods, we naturally would combine the objectives derived from consideration of patients' needs with other objectives which would make the program properly student-centered. Hence the student nurse learns to meet the patients' needs. The outcome is a student who has learned, and patients who benefit because there is a continuing supply of graduate nurses to give direct care to patients. Let me illustrate. I believe the patient in the hospital is entitled to nursing care which will complement and supplement the medical care plan in such a way as to produce maximum benefit for the patient. I believe the nursing service should provide the basic supportive care necessary for physical and emotional comfort, rest, safety, and hygiene for all patients. I believe that nursing service should help the patient move positively from dependency to the maximum degree of independent activity consistent with his medical condition.

I believe the hospital patient and his family are entitled to know what care the patient needs after discharge, and be taught whatever is necessary to encourage maximum recovery, prevent further illness, and attain the best possible adjustment in the family. I believe the patient is entitled to such care regardless of who gives the care. The nurse guiding the auxiliary workers, therefore, has an obligation, and so she should be prepared to teach the worker and supplement the auxiliary care to make these goals possible for the patient. The degree of comprehensiveness will depend on the patient's needs. Not every patient needs, nor wants, the same care.

Now what does this mean for the nurse graduating from a diploma program? Is what I have described just technical education? Do we need or want just technicians to give this care? Of course the nurse must have tools with which to work—mental and physical. If our objectives in nursing care are the same, they can be formulated by a study of the goals of the patient care program. Neither objectives nor tools can be adopted verbatim from my plan, from the National League for Nursing list, or any other piece of literature. Patient care goals will enable the faculty to adapt such materials to their own plan. Wisely adapted, they will be helpful objectives and useful tools.

In the preparation of a nurse for direct patient care, the tools of health and home care are included because the patient and family must be taught so that the patient may care for himself at home—not because the faculty wish or intend to prepare the diploma graduate for work in public health nursing. Students in the diploma program learn how to make a referral to the visiting nurse service because continuity of care for the patient when he returns home may be a significant factor in determining whether he gets well and stays well—not because they are to work in the community as public health nurses. Included also are elements of administration, because these are an essential part of good planning, and good planning produces more effective care, is more economical of learning time, and more satisfying to a future worker—not because a head nurse or supervisor is being prepared. The elements of problem solving will be included, because good care of people involves identification of problems and ability to marshal pertinent facts and select the most appropriate solution—not because the basic course prepares its graduates to do studies and research. This is all on the level of a student with the background of sciences and nursing which can be given appropriately in a hospital diploma program, and used by the graduate of such a program in her care of patients.

I believe we directors of diploma programs are much to blame for our present confusion. We have not spoken with clarity or conviction. Too often we are inclined to copy another program, instead of studying and devising our own. Too often we have sought change because the League required it— not because it was right. We have wanted too much for our graduates. We have worked hard, but sometimes toward unrealistic goals. Because our plans were inadequate, or unsound, or not well adapted to our particular situation, we have had a sense of failure, or frustration, or inadequacy. We have lost faith in ourselves and the future of the diploma school.

We in diploma schools need today, almost more than ever before, some of the fresh, energetic qualities of a child to combine with our maturity of insight. We need to believe in belief. We need to be humble enough to listen to the little voices—the patients. We don't need to perform miracles, but we do need to take what is before us and make it fit our situation so that we may move forward. We need to seek out our fairy godmother, not always outside ourselves or our educational systems, but from within.

We have the support of our hospitals and medical staffs if we will help them understand our dilemmas and our needs. We have the possibility, if we will hold on to it and use it, of leadership from NLN. We have the privilege of sharing our gains in our own Council of Diploma and Associate Degree Programs. With this we can, if we will, prepare the necessary quantity and quality of nurses to assure the American people the direct nursing care they need.

It is time for all of us together to make a statement of our belief in the diploma school for all to use—our own schools, our hospitals, and our communities. Once this is done, we must then study our situations to learn how best to move constructively toward improvement in the diploma school in which we have together reaffirmed our belief.

Tentative Statement of Belief in Diploma Programs

The NLN's Council of Member Agencies of the Department of Diploma and Associate Degree Programs, at its meeting in Atlantic City in June, approved the revised tentative statement of belief pertaining to educational programs in nursing leading to a diploma and referred it to the department's steering committee and NLN board for further action. This statement has since been approved by the steering committee, and action by the NLN board and membership is pending:

Nursing in its broad scope is a profession that employs persons with varying degrees of ability and preparation. There is a need for educational programs designed to prepare these persons. In order to assist in maintaining and increasing the number of registered nurses required to meet the expanding demands for nursing services, the NLN believes that educationally sound diploma programs in nursing offered by independent or hospital controlled schools are essential.

Such diploma programs offer education in nursing which prepares graduates for general duty nursing positions in hospitals, nursing homes, and comparable situations and form a basis for further study and specialization if desired. Graduates of these programs are prepared to function as specified in the current criteria to utilize the understandings and to demonstrate the personal characteristics outline therein.*

The NLN believes that graduates of diploma programs, like other graduate nurses, when exposed to new and complex situations, should be thoroughly oriented through in-service education.

* National League for Nursing. *Criteria for the Evaluation of Educational Programs in Nursing Leading to a Diploma.* New York: The League, 1958, pp. 18–22.

Nursing education is still in the process of change. The next decade or so will perhaps be decisive in determining which direction nursing education will take. The problem was emphasized by the Surgeon General's Consultant Group on Nursing.

8.

The Continuing Problems in Nursing Education

Major changes in the practice and concepts of medicine are extending the scope of health services. Hospitals are giving increasingly complex care to a greater number of patients. Skilled nursing care homes are growing in number. Communities are developing more and better outpatient services and home-care programs for the mentally as well as the physically ill. Medical science confers more benefits than ever before and new achievements come at a rapid rate.

At the same time, sociological and economic trends are magnifying de-

From *Toward Quality in Nursing: Needs and Goals.* Report of the Surgeon Generals' Consultant Group on Nursing, Public Health Publication No. 992, U. S. Department of Health, Education, and Welfare, 1963, pp. 54–57.

mands for service. Between 1960 and 1970 the population of the United States will increase at a rate equivalent to adding each year a city the size of Chicago, with the proportion of older people and babies on the rise. The people of the United States are becoming better educated and more sophisticated about health and medical care, and are seeking in various ways to lessen the financial barriers to adequate health services, including nursing care.

The demands of the future will soar. Yet the United States does not now have enough adequately trained nurses to meet today's most pressing needs for care. With 550,000 professional nurses in practice in 1962, most institutions and areas had serious shortages of staff. In many places the quality of care has suffered as inadequately prepared nurses and inadequately trained auxiliary personnel have had to provide care beyond their capacity. In 1962 the total number of practical nurses and auxiliary workers employed— 225,000 practical nurses and over 400,000 aides, orderlies, and attendants— exceeded the total number of professional nurses.

Although responsibilities of professional nurses have constantly increased as the complexity of medical care has grown, not enough nurses receive the strong educational background necessary for positions of leadership. Most professional nurses are still being prepared in hospital diploma programs. Too few nurses come from the baccalaureate programs—4-year collegiate programs offering stronger foundations in science and a broader perspective of the liberal arts. Even fewer receive graduate education for teaching, supervisory, administrative, and specialized clinical positions.

Looking ahead, nursing personnel should contribute to the health services of the Nation in a way now possible in only a few institutions and areas. More nurses will be needed to engage in the highly skilled care of hospital patients and in the administration and supervision of hospital nursing services. The mentally ill inside and outside hospitals should receive care from specially prepared nurses. Strengthened nursing home and school and public health services will require more well-trained nurses. More nurse teachers must help educate future generations of nurses.

To give the people of the United States safe, therapeutically effective, and efficient nursing service, some 850,000 professional nurses and 350,000 practical nurses would be needed by 1970. But to meet this need would require a total of 100,000 graduates of basic professional nursing schools a year beginning in 1966—a tripling of the present output of a little over 30,000. In view of limited school capacity and recruitment problems, a realistic goal would be to increase the number of graduates to 53,000 a year by 1969. With this increase there should be a total of some 680,000 nurses in 1970.

There must be a major expansion of both diploma and collegiate programs to increase the number of professional nurse graduates from 30,000 to 53,000. Large financial investment will be required for this purpose. Special emphasis must be given to the basic baccalaureate degree programs. These must double their graduates, from the 1960 level of 4,000 to a total of at least 8,000 in 1970. This expansion will probably require the establishment of 30 or more new collegiate nursing schools.

Many more well-qualified candidates must be attracted into nursing, particularly from among the college-bound. Opportunities in nursing must be more vigorously publicized by schools; communities; State, regional, and national organizations; and government agencies. We must increase the recruitment pool by greater emphasis on minority groups, men, and older and married women. Programs of financial aid to students will be essential to attract young people who cannot now afford education beyond high school. Finally, to attract and hold the needed nursing personnel, salaries and economic benefits for nursing must come nearer to equalling those of other occupations requiring comparable preparation, ability, and responsibility.

Advanced preparation of nurses for leadership and teaching positions must receive greater emphasis and support. This will require expansion and development of new programs for graduate education. Additional short-term training programs will also be needed. More graduates of diploma programs must be given an opportunity to return to school to gain more scientific knowledge.

We must take a more critical look at patterns of nursing education. A broad study of the whole complex of currently unrelated educational programs for nursing should be undertaken to determine how nursing schools might better keep pace with technological and scientific advances. Such a study would require a 5- to 10-year effort. It should have broad professional participation, under the leadership of the nursing profession.

For the immediate future, present nursing education programs must be more strongly supported, expanded, and improved. This will require thorough regional, State, and community appraisal of nursing education needs. It will demand construction of costly teaching facilities, as well as more and better-prepared faculty and the development of new educational methods.

Maximum service must be obtained from existing nursing personnel. To make the best use of nursing skills now available, there must be substantial improvement in hospital and nursing administration and in nursing staff assignments. There must be careful and widespread studies of the present utilization of personnel, and more experimentation with nursing staffing patterns.

Continuous staff education is equally necessary for high quality nursing service. This must include inservice education for professional and practical nurses, on-the-job training for nursing aides, and continuing education outside the employing institution. These staff education programs should be primarily supported by the health institutions themselves, but aid is needed to promote their development.

Nursing research must be stimulated. Research in nursing has just begun to yield the body of knowledge needed as a basis for the improvement of patient care. Support is urgently needed for research in relatively untouched areas. Much greater support is required for patient-oriented studies in line with changing patterns of patient care.

No one group in the Nation will be able to accomplish all of these purposes. The nursing profession, other health professions, community groups, foundations, private philanthropists, colleges and universities, and hospitals are among the groups which will need to cooperate in the effort to meet nursing service requirements in years to come. Where these groups lack the necessary financial and technical resources to meet minimum goals, governments at all levels must provide appropriate support. A share of the responsibility must be borne by the Federal Government.

In accordance with the Surgeon General's charge to the Consultant Group, the specific recommendations of this report are directed to the areas in which Federal assistance can be of particular and immediate significance in increasing and improving nursing personnel and nursing service. Those recommendations, which have been discussed in some detail in chapters VI to X, are repeated as the conclusion of this chapter.

We wish first, however, to emphasize our urgent recommendation to the nursing profession:

Study of nursing education. A study should be made of the present system of nursing education in relation to the responsibilities and skill levels required for high-quality patient care. This study should be started immediately so that nursing education programs can benefit as soon as possible from the findings. Funds for such a study should be obtained from private and government sources.

The Consultant Group recommends to the Surgeon General of the Public Health Service that the Federal Government substantially expand and add to its present program of support and assistance to nursing and nursing education. Specifically:

Stimulation of recruitment to schools of nursing. The Public Health Service should expand its efforts and give financial and other assistance to

State, regional, and national agencies for recruitment programs for nursing and other health personnel.

Federal funds should be made available to schools of professional nursing and of practical nursing approved by agencies designated by the Surgeon General of the Public Health Service, to enable them to offer low-cost loans, cancelable in part by a specified number of years of full-time employment in nursing, to eligible or enrolled students who show reasonable promise of success in nursing and who can provide evidence of financial need.

Federal funds should be made available to provide scholarships to attract a greater number of highly qualified high school graduates who need financial assistance into collegiate programs of nursing which are nationally approved by agencies designated by the Surgeon General of the Public Health Service.

Assistance to schools of nursing to expand and improve the quality of educational programs. Federal funds should be provided to help meet the construction needs for educational facilities for schools of nursing.

Federal funds should be made available for grants to institutions, regional, State and other public and nonprofit organizations or agencies for planning and determining the need for new nursing school facilities or new, expanded, or improved programs of nursing education.

Federal funds for planning grants for construction of nursing education facilities should be made available to universities, colleges and schools of professional nursing which are ready to expand or establish new schools of nursing.

Steps should be taken by the Public Health Service and the nursing profession to prepare prototypes of school facilities most conducive to efficient and effective teaching of nursing.

Federal funds should be made available, by means of project grants, to nursing education programs in universities, colleges, schools, and in public and nonprofit hospitals, institutions, and agencies—for the improvement, expansion, and extension of their educational programs and services. This would include experimentation with the demonstration of new and effective methods of teaching, the development and use of teaching aids and equipment, and, where indicated, the establishment of new programs.

Federal funds should be made available to reimburse schools of nursing for partial costs of education of students supported wholly or in part by Federal scholarships or loans.

Assistance to professional nurses for advanced training. The present Federal programs of Professional Nurse Traineeships administered by the Public Health Service should be extended and gradually increased to at least double (within a 5-year period) the present number of full time trainees. The duration of the traineeship should be extended to cover the period prescribed for the individual trainee to complete the program of study. In the administration of the program greater emphasis should be given to the support of candidates for the doctoral degree.

The Professional Nurse Traineeship Program should be expanded to provide for preparation of nursing specialists in clinical fields.

The present funds for short-term training in the Professional Nurse Traineeship Program should be doubled immediately and increased as needed thereafter; these increases should in no way reduce funds appropriated for full-time traineeships.

Federal funds should be provided for traineeships for nurse graduates of diploma and associate degree programs for up to 2 years of full-time study toward a baccalaureate degree. Eligibility should be limited to nurses who entered diploma or associate degree programs prior to inception of this traineeship program. During the first year of the program, funds should be made available to about 1 percent of the diploma and associate degree graduates now practicing. The number of trainees should be increased in succeeding years.

Federal funds should be provided to compensate the schools taking part in the Professional Nurse Traineeship Program to cover partial costs of education of the trainees.

Assistance to hospitals and health agencies to improve the utilization and training of nursing personnel. Federal funds should be made available to improve the utilization of nursing service personnel by providing project grants for demonstrations, for experimentation with new and improved methods, and for training in use of these methods. State and other public and nonprofit institutions, organizations, and agencies should be eligible for these grants.

Additional funds should be made available to expand those Public Health Service programs which provide consultation and other services to hospitals and other health institutions and agencies to improve the quality and quantity of patient care through better utilization of nursing service personnel and other appropriate methods.

Federal funds should be made available by means of project grants to nursing schools and other appropriate agencies, as determined by the Surgeon General of the Public Health Service, for strengthening inservice education, on-the-job training, and continuing education to help nursing service personnel improve their nursing knowledge and skills.

Increased support for research. Funds for the Nursing Research Fellowship Program of the Public Health Service should be increased to provide immediately for 100 new full-time research fellowships. This number should be increased as additional qualified nurses apply.

Funds for the Public Health Service intramural program of research in nursing should be doubled with future increases as the need arises.

Funds for the Public Health Service program of extramural research grants in nursing should be substantially increased. The increase should provide for a larger number of research grants and support more varied types of investigations. More consultation on nursing research methodology should be provided by the Public Health Service, and schools of nursing should be eligible for research development grants.

II NURSING AS A PROFESSION

American society has been defined as a society of professionals. Talcott Parsons, one of America's leading sociologists, has said that one of the distinguishing marks of modern society has been the emergence of so many different professional groups. But what is a profession, and is nursing a profession? Most authorities would agree that belonging to a profession implies an aspiration towards a certain status in society. This status would include licensure, an identification of the activities of the group with the public interest, the establishment of codes related to the conduct of the members, and a consciousness on the part of the members of being part of a profession. A profession should be an intellectual operation that puts great reliance upon individual responsibility, and it should have practical application, a tendency towards self-organization, a growing body of knowledge, and a technique that can be taught. The professional stance in relation to clients is marked by a code of values that stresses altruistic behavior. By these criteria, nursing can be called a profession, but unfortunately it is more a profession in some respects than in others. Therefore, professional recognition for nursing depends upon how the criteria are further refined, and what particular aspects are emphasized.

Eli Ginzberg who headed a national study on the role of nurses in modern society (*A Program for the Nursing Profession,* by the Committee on the Function of Nursing, The Macmillan Co., 1948), has been most critical of the attempts of nurses to claim professional status. In the extract which follows, Dr. Ginzberg goes so far as to claim that nursing is not a profession and could not become one until fundamental changes take place.

9.

Nursing Is Not A Profession

Dr. Eli Ginzberg, the speaker, paused and looked at me. "I hope you understand that I'm a friend of nurses," he said. "You're a fine group and you're doing good work. But I have to state facts as I see them.

"Your trouble is that you're misclassifying yourselves. And as an economist, I can tell you that's bad practice in the labor market. You seldom gain in salary or status, and you often lose."

"Suppose," I suggested, "that we nurses accepted your viewpoint. What then? Do you mean we should reclassify ourselves?"

"Yes, I do. But to be sure we don't get mixed up in a word game, let's first define the word *profession*. To me it means a group that 1) has broad training, 2) provides recognized intellectual leadership in its field, 3) does significant research, and 4) is independent enough to define its own area of work.

"Now, if we accept this definition, then I suggest the following:

"First, call your nurses who are graduates of the two- and three-year schools *technicians*. After all, there's nothing indecent about being a good technician. Nobody thinks poorly of the electrician or the TV repair man, and *they're* doing well in the labor market.

"Then, start developing a much more delimited group—graduates of *good* college or university programs—that you can properly call *professional* nurses.

"*Now* is a good time to do your planning for this change. The population is increasing rapidly. The medical profession already is hard put to maintain an adequate ratio of physicians. And, in my opinion, the supply of doctors in proportion to the population will shrink as time goes on.

"So, medicine will have to start (and is starting) to restudy and reassign many of its duties. Here's a golden opportunity for professional nurses to become, in effect, junior doctors.

"But note this: Nurses will have to be prepared to handle this assignment through proper education and experience. *They must first become professionals.*"

"Just why," I asked, "do you think we aren't *now* professionals?"

"For several reasons. First, much of your education lacks the breadth—the development of general understanding and critical awareness—that education for a profession tends to give one.

From an interview, "Is Nursing Really a Profession?" by Patricia D. Horgan. Reprinted by permission from *RN* Magazine. Copyright January and February 1960, RN Publications, Inc., Oradell, N. J.

"Your three-year diploma program started as a means of making it easy for a girl to 1) pay her own way while 2) giving service and while 3) learning a few fundamentals! It was also a means for the hospital—always hard-pressed financially—to get nurses at a cost it could afford. That was fine at the time. But it didn't—and doesn't—produce a *professional* person.

"Can you imagine doctors, lawyers, engineers—or school teachers!—getting their training this way? In the old days, yes. But not for many decades. Today the members of professions get their education within the accepted framework of a college or a university."

"But," I objected, "we *do* have college nursing programs."

"Granted. But you won't be a profession until *all* your nursing programs are under the direction of colleges and universities.

"My second point has to do with the nature of your present college programs. I get the impression that you're putting too much emphasis on preparing nurses to become administrators.

"Now, it's all right to educate some people for administration *if* administration is related to important functions of the profession.

"But I think your stress on administration pushes aside the education you should be giving for what you *do*—in other words, for the *practice* of nursing. Your higher education should deal with nursing practice and procedures more scientifically than it does at present. It should delve more deeply into such subjects as the social and emotional needs of the patient. And it should concern itself more broadly with background subjects—for instance, chemistry, physiology, and the like."

Dr. Ginzberg paused. "My third point is closely related to this," he went on. "In a profession part of the leadership is constantly doing research that improves professional theory and practice. There's a lively intellectual development going on.

"Most of the members don't take part in this. But there's a place at the top for those who do. And they have the backing of the profession at large.

"This isn't true in nursing. It *is* true that improvements are being made in technical and administrative procedures. But there's not much research about the theory behind nursing practice.

"Now to my fourth point: A profession has a certain independence that allows it to redefine and modify its work. Nursing doesn't have this. Basically, it's still an appendage of medicine; and here's why:

"Liberally defined, the nurse's education—not counting her hours in non-academic work—equals about a year of college study. The doctor has seven to eight years of college and medical school, plus one year of internship. That's eight to nine years compared to one! And a specialist has several years of additional study.

"Now, what happens when a decision is needed that concerns a patient? Logically, the person with eight or more years of preparation makes it," he said, "not the person with one year.

"Here, I believe, is the reason nurses are self-conscious about being 'professionals.' They realize this tremendous gap exists.

"For my final point, let's consider the number of active nurses (now at about 460,000, I understand). Because you're such a large group, it's difficult for you to develop as a clearly defined profession. And, economically, it's impossible for you to be paid at a professional level—especially since your group keeps growing larger all the time.

"As I see it, you nurses face a sort of economic-bootstrap dilemma. Without the pay, you can't attract the well-trained people you need to raise the level of skill. And without raising the level of skill, you can't command professional pay!

"This is where you stand at the moment. And this is why, I suspect, so many of your nurses with degrees go into administration or teaching. These are practically the only positions offering added pay for broader training.

"You've asked," said Dr. Eli Ginzberg, "for a definition of nursing at what I consider a professional level. Let me answer by giving my concept of the truly professional nurse.

"She'll be a top-level practitioner with more authority than today's nurse. Her relationship with the doctor will be similar to, say, the relationship between the general practitioner and the specialist. In other words, she'll have a voice in controlling the moves affecting her patient.

"For example, I can see a nurse with advanced training and experience in surgery making the observations and recommendations on which the surgeon will base his decision whether to operate, and when to operate. And after the operation—the doctor having made his initial visit and outlined the post-op care—I can see the nurse taking over responsibility for such things as dressings and the management of fluids."

"This," I said, "is what many nurses would *like* to see happen. But we're realists. We can't see the doctor sharing his authority in this way."

"In some areas, he has already begun to share it," said Dr. Ginzberg. "Take psychiatry, for example. In many institutions, a large part of what psychiatrists are doing is based on the recommendations of nurses who are in constant contact with the patients.

"And why do these psychiatrists act on the nurses' recommendations? For two reasons: 1) They recognize their nurses as competent specialists. 2) They just can't keep in close contact, personally, with their many patients. So they *have to* rely on the nurses, who can.

"As time goes on, population growth will get so far ahead of the doctors that, like today's institutional psychiatrists, they'll become swamped. They'll have to turn over decision-making in more, and broader, areas of patient-care. But they'll insist that before they release authority, those who would receive it must be experts in their field.

"The nurse deals with the patient's total needs. So she'll have to have a sound knowledge indeed before the doctor will hand over a large share of the decision-making about his patient!"

"That explains your opinion that we need to improve our educational programs before we can become professionals," I said. "Now what other steps do you believe we should take?"

Dr. Ginzberg paused. "First," he said, "you'll want to restudy the nurses' work as it relates to the physicians' work. You'll want to decide—with the cooperation of the medical profession—exactly what work can be done by a group of superior nurses.

"Then you'll select these first professional nurses from your present ranks. (There won't be many of them at first.) You'll pick nurses who are outstandingly competent because of 1) natural talent, 2) a high level of academic and clinical training, and 3) a record of exceptional performance.

"You'll promote recognition for these nurses among other nurses and doctors. You'll help them get assignments appropriate to their skills.

"Second, you'll set up standards for your new corps of professionals. You'll mold the standards to fit the kinds of jobs that are open, or are likely to be open. You'll designate the kind and amount of education required.

"Third, you'll recruit and educate only the number of professional nurses you think are needed. Economically, this last point is very important. Only by limiting your group to, say, a top figure of 70,000 can you hope to get professional pay.

"Now, let's suppose you've started this elite corps. Your next step is to face the fact, frankly, that there are some 800,000 to 1,000,000 men and women in the business of patient-care.

"When you do, you'll recognize—as many nurses already recognize— that those outside the ranks of R.N.s are co-workers, not competitors. You'll recognize that it's proper to use some of them at certain levels of work after a short period of job training. You'll recognize that still others can function well at higher levels after a longer period of work *and* study.

"Finally, you'll see yourselves—the present R.N.—in true perspective. You'll proudly recognize that the R.N. is the key to the future progress of those below and the new group above. For those below look up to her for advice and training. And many of the new professionals come from her ranks.

"I believe that while you're thinking this through, you'll recognize that nurses with two to three years' *training* (as opposed to *education*) are, rightly speaking, technicians. You'll start thinking of them as technicians. But your pride in them won't change. For you'll know that good technicians are respected by everyone.

"When you've arrived at this viewpoint, I think you'll quit fighting futile battles about status. Instead, you'll concentrate on developing your professional group. And you'll see to it that avenues are left open so that everyone of ambition and ability—from the newest aide to the most experienced R.N. —can move toward the top.

"Let me illustrate: Many of today's teachers, lawyers, and engineers started their working lives as, say, clerk-typists, salesmen, and factory workers. But they went to night school while they worked or took time off for college. And when they became qualified, the professions they had prepared for accepted them."

Dr. Ginzberg paused again, then concluded: "One final word of caution: From what I've seen, you nurses tend to go off by yourselves to try to solve your problems. Don't tackle *this* problem on your own or you may never manage to lift yourselves to a professional level!

"The advances I've been talking about will come *only* after a tremendous amount of cooperative effort. You'll need to enlist the help of hospital administrators, of educators, and—above all—of doctors. Once you have these friends on your side, you can move ahead with excellent chances for success."

Professor Ginzberg's negative portrayal of the professional status of the nurse is somewhat contradicted by the more hopeful picture given by Genevieve and Roy Bixler. This husband and wife team first examined the professional aspects of nursing in 1945, and then studied them again in 1959 to find if nursing had changed. They found that nursing had indeed taken some steps to improve its professional status, but they found several areas in which nursing did not measure up to the criteria that they utilized.

10.

The Professional Status of Nursing

by Genevieve K. Bixler and Roy W. Bixler

1. A profession utilizes in its practice a well-defined and well-organized body of specialized knowledge which is on the intellectual level of the higher learning.

To what extent has nursing advanced in utilizing a body of knowledge peculiarly its own which is on the intellectual level of the higher learning?

Some progress can be noted since this criterion was studied in 1945. There was for a time, beginning about 10 years ago, some recognition in the nursing literature of the need to identify scientific principles peculiar to nursing and to experiment with new science courses in 2-, 3-, and 4-year basic nursing programs. More recently this interest appears to have declined, for it is not being referred to in descriptions of school curriculums, nor on programs of curriculum conferences, nor in other activities which normally reveal the live interests and concerns of nurse educators. It may be that the testing of such courses now occupies the educators and that soon the outcomes will be ready for more general consideration. On the other hand, it is possible that this idea, so vigorously promoted a few years ago, now seems less essential.

There has been a decided trend toward employing faculties of junior and liberal arts colleges for the science instruction commonly concentrated in the first and second years of nursing programs. For the most part, the nursing student has adapted to these science teachers and their courses rather than the reverse. We have talked about the value to the nursing student of association in such courses with students of other interests on the campus. Including nursing students in these science courses has freed some nurse educators for other kinds of instruction, and it has provided students with instructors who have had more preparation in specific science areas than most nurse science instructors have had. Does this satisfy the first criterion, or is there still great need for study and experimentation of the elements of science uniquely underlying the practice of nursing? This is a question that seems not to have been faced squarely by nursing educators.

Willingness to undergo long-time examination of scientific principles, discussion within groups of imaginative, flexible science professors and nurse educators, and experimentation with new organizations of science content continue to seem as essential at this time as they were considered

Reprinted, with permission, from *The American Journal of Nursing*, LIX 1959, 1142–1147.

to be years ago. General courses in science for college students not planning to major in science might include only the most basic principles from physics, chemistry, microbiology, biochemistry, and other science fields—principles newly formulated so as to break down the present barriers between science specialties. If several colleges could stay with such efforts for a few years of rigorous experimentation, they might demonstrate that time could be saved and learning enhanced for students who need such a science base though they do not plan for careers in fields of pure science.

Now, how does this relate to nursing? If, as has been suggested, general science courses should form the introduction of many college students to the application of scientific principles within their own fields, then nurse scientists would need to continue to supply the science instruction in nursing at the next level. With such a foundation, nursing students could then be ready to assimilate the scientific principles unique to nursing. If, as we say, the teaching in our better nursing programs today focuses upon the *why* instead of the *how*, we are already teaching an applied science of nursing. This can be much improved, with a reduction of duplication, as the various clinical fields themselves become less rigidly compartmentalized.

Today's best qualified clinical instructors promise to be tomorrow's teachers of nursing science. Some bright young scholars might be encouraged to undertake the study of nursing science at least to the level of a doctor's degree, so there could be thorough testing of the ways in which present-day science instruction and clinical instruction might be associated more closely. And all who are preparing to be clinical instructors should have a better orientation to the scientific principles underlying clinical content.

One additional observation may safely be made at this point. There is considerable evidence of progress in recent years in the contributions of the behavioral sciences to nursing. This seems to have been due in great part to the willingness, even eagerness, of many behavioral scientists to adapt their materials to the needs of nursing and nursing education. Many contributions from general courses in these fields have been incorporated in nursing programs in recent years.

2. A profession constantly enlarges the body of knowledge it uses and improves its techniques of education and service by the use of the scientific method.

The so-called research function of a profession constitutes this second criterion. Nursing has made much progress in the past 14 years in the extension of its body of knowledge, systematically derived, and in its dependence upon the scientific method rather than upon the jury method of ascertaining truths. There is considerable evidence to support this assertion.

For some time the national nursing organizations have supported research by encouragement, by planning, and by subsidy. The National League of Nursing Education and its successor, the National League for Nursing, have sponsored much study relating to the education of nurses. They have also stimulated study by many individuals through dissemination of historical and bibliographical materials, and through conferences in which planning and reporting of studies take place. This organization has emphasized particularly curriculums of schools of nursing.

The American Nurses' Association has stimulated much action research in recent years. Its growing interest was shown in June 1958 by the highly significant action of the ANA House of Delegates, which unanimously adopted research as its number one long-term goal: "[To] stimulate efforts by nurses and other specialists to identify and enlarge the scientific principle upon which nursing rests, and to encourage research by them in the application of these principles to nursing."

The establishment of the American Nurses' Foundation by the ANA in 1955 represents a significant advance in the area of research. Although its work is in the initial stages, its incorporation is an important index of the growth of nursing toward full professional status. The Foundation is chartered to increase the public knowledge and understanding of professional and practical nursing and of the science and arts upon which the health of the American people depends, by engaging in studies, surveys, and research, and through research grants to public and private nonprofit educational institutions. As a matter of policy, the Foundation has a special interest in supporting research and educational projects in areas of need not met by other sources.

With this incorporation, the American Nurses' Association transferred to the Foundation its responsibility for administering a program of research in nursing, under which it had distributed $285,390 in a 4-year period, funds which came directly from ANA members. Since the Foundation's incorporation, it has received funds from other sources, because of its tax-free status, and it has distributed in grants a total of $105,835 for 10 projects in five states and the District of Columbia. In addition to these, the Foundation staff is carrying on projects in three areas of needed research which were not covered by other proposals submitted. These projects are being supported by the National Institutes of Health and the Rockefeller Foundation.

Extending its support of research, the American Nurses' Foundation conducted a conference in September 1958 to which were invited representatives of many institutions and agencies who have either been doing research in nursing or promoting it. This 3-day conference at Western Reserve University enabled about 100 individuals, chiefly nurses, to discuss mutual research interests and make some future plans which seem likely to produce further progress in nursing. Such a conference could not have taken place profitably a decade ago.

Progress in research is manifest in another area. A few years ago the Southern Regional Education Board sought support to establish a research institute for the centralization of research functions in connection with regional programs of graduate study in nursing. Failure to obtain support readily for this institute resulted in a re-examination of the concept, and then a slower and much less dramatic plan evolved. The objective is now to stimulate larger numbers of graduate nursing students who may only be beginning to develop some competence in the conduct and administration of research.

As a result of this plan, many nurses in the South now have a new concept of the place of research in their programs and a beginning competence in use of research methods. Through the limited skills developed in the first year of graduate study, some promising masters' theses have been produced. An effort has been made to bring some of these together as cooperative research, and the results are demonstrating that well-planned small pieces of research may be coordinated which jointly produce more useful knowledge than can be developed by individuals working separately.

The newer concept of endeavoring to involve more individuals in the varied activities of research, instead of having a few working for the many, is a more democratic one than a superimposed arrangement. Moreover, as the products of undergraduate collegiate and graduate programs in nursing increase in number and influence, the production, interpretation, and utilization of research seems likely to increase in amount and value. In spite of the significant advances, much now presented as research in nursing has been of limited value in advancing the frontiers of knowledge in the health professions.

Research has little use if the findings are not disseminated. For many years the *American Journal of Nursing* carried the major burden of informing all groups of nurses on all aspects of the profession. Now the American Journal of Nursing Company publishes two other periodicals, serving varied purposes and extending the coverage. *Nursing Outlook,* first published in 1953, began as interpreter of the newly organized National League for Nursing. Analysis of the contents of *Nursing Outlook* in the years since it was founded shows with what faithfulness it has hewed to the concept of its function as stated in the first issue of the magazine. Through its reporting, *Nursing Outlook* has extended nursing literature appreciably, and has made slow but steady growth in the reading public it has reached.

More dramatic, however, has been the appearance on the journalistic scene of *Nursing Research,* begun in June 1952, and dedicated to the reporting and dissemination of research in nursing. Now published four times a year, it has reported a variety of studies and much news about research. The periodical is small and has not yet begun to support itself by its own list of subscribers. Nevertheless, it is making a contribution to research in nursing not previously possible.

Research is also being better supported in other ways. Through the subsidy of foundations, some manufacturing concerns, the U.S. Public Health Service, and occasionally an individual, research has received a great deal of encouragement. Within the scope of this article it is impossible to list the many studies that have brought new knowledge to the nursing profession.

3. A profession entrusts the education of its practitioners to institutions of higher education.

Utilization of the resources of higher education for professional preparation of the practitioners of nursing is growing slowly. There has been an increase since 1945 in the number of schools offering preparation for nursing within the framework of higher education, and also in the number of students enrolled in such programs. Considering the expansion of collegiate education since the end of World War II, the expansion in nursing education is not remarkable, however.

Significant development has been the increase in the number of graduate programs in nursing. Though increase in number of schools and even in number of students is by no means the only criterion of improvement, the greater supply of better prepared teachers, administrators, and service-responsible nurses cannot fail to improve nursing as a profession. The greatly increased number of scholarships and fellowships for nursing students is also contributing to the profession's advancement through greater use of higher education.

It is difficult to discuss this criterion separately, for more education and better earning power, as well as the improved social and political position of women, have all contributed to the forward march of nurses. There can now be no doubt that by their competence, their dependability, and their devotion to duty, the nurses who had military service in World War II exemplified something beyond any earlier appreciation of the role of this group in the world's affairs. It was fortunate for nursing that the G.I. Bill of Rights recognized this professional group. Many nurses owe their opportunity to do advanced study, some all the way to the doctor's degree, to the fact that they served in the uniform of their country.

The genesis in 1954 of a regional project for nursing education on the graduate level was another significant development and one which reflected the improved professional status of nursing. This successful experiment in cooperative planning for graduate education in nursing in 16 states has been under the sponsorship of the Southern Regional Education Board. Though the current phase of this project nears an end, the cooperating universities will continue their programs, and new projects are forming from the momentum of the past five years. Now, the Western Interstate Commission for Higher Education has initiated a second regional project which is also demonstrating the concern of higher education for improved preparation of nursing instructors, administrators, and service-oriented nurses.

4. A profession applies its body of knowledge in practical services which are vital to human and social welfare.

Though much of the world today lives by humanitarian principles and practices, we are being increasingly dominated by considerations of such baleful import as to cause many to doubt the ability of the human race to survive. In the midst of the traditional image of the nurse as the "angel of mercy," she must also be viewed as a key figure in disaster nursing. This is less the merciful figure easing the hurts of the wounded and closing the eyes of the dying than the highly skilled administrator of block action who expedites treatment of the least severely damaged inhabitants and moves the, as yet, uninjured away from contaminated areas. Can nurses play these opposing roles if need arises? Probably so. Without dwelling upon this nightmare prospect, we should go on to examine the extension of the traditional humanitarian role.

At the end of World War II the United States enjoyed great prestige abroad as the greatest military power in the world and, in the next few years, as the friend of many tottering small (and not so small) nations newly striving for political and economic survival. Nurses were on the highly professional teams representing our government which went into remote places to bring healing, better nutrition, sanitation, education, and economic soundness to the less fortunate people of the world. The prestige which these nurses built for their profession was of a very high order.

The profession has continued the trend to ever higher concepts of service, and the high reputation for such service, both at home and abroad. Willingness to offer a few years of service out of the mainstream of a promising career continues to show in the increased numbers of competent nurses who accept a term in some remote region, thus sacrificing tenure, advancement, and greater remuneration at home, in order to serve the more basic needs of society.

It is well known that the government of the United States has not maintained its high esteem abroad, so the position of today's nurses is the more significant. In the several international organizations whose programs are now very familiar to all who read and listen, the American nurses and the organizations they represent play an increasingly effective role. We are assured that in the highest circles of our government, nurses are invited as participants for many more occasions than was the case a few years ago. Nurses, in ever greater numbers, are taking a place in planning and doing the work of the world. There has come about almost a complete change from the reluctance and self-effacing attitudes of some years ago to an eagerness and quiet assumption of confidence now betokening professional equality with other and older professions.

5. A profession functions autonomously in the formulation of professional policy and in the control of professional activity thereby.

This criterion needs some clarification. Functioning autonomously refers to the positions of schools within the framework of education and in relation to government structure. A school of nursing, to be autonomous, should be independent of control by any other professional school or agency. It is also a general rule that in matters affecting a profession it is that profession which interprets its needs and goals and takes leadership in presenting the ways such needs may be met and the goals attained. Of course, a profession welcomes the ideas and suggestions of allied professional groups, especially in attacking problems in which there are common goals.

In time now largely past, nursing had difficulty being permitted the professional courtesy of self-determination, mainly because nursing was thought of as serving doctors and as being apprenticed to medicine. The brief period of schooling, plus the nature of the activities nurses were allowed to engage in, also contributed to the subservient relationship. Such factors as the lengthening period of preparation for nursing, the more democratic attitude of many physicians and related team workers, and the increased responsibilities which nurses have proved they can assume, have led to greater freedom for nursing in the determination of its own goals and the means to achieve them.

The work of all eight sections of the ANA in the development of functions, standards, and qualifications has been an important step in the direction of professional autonomy. Nurses have defined their own functions and the standards which should govern the quality of their service. The very assumption of this prerogative is an index of professional status.

Unfortunately, there is resistance to higher standards that accompany the advance of nursing toward full professional status, and this resistance comes not alone from individuals in other professional groups. Efforts to upgrade the profession are resisted by nurses themselves, albeit a small group. Naturally enough, this minority appears to be made up of representatives of some of the weaker schools and of practicing nurses with less adequate preparation to cope with present-day demands on the profession. To abet such a resistance to improved standards, representatives of other professions sometimes lend support, especially if they seem likely to gain certain benefits for their own group or institutions.

The movement by representatives of some of the unaccredited 3-year programs against nationwide accreditation seems shortsighted and contrary to the trend toward professionalization. While many 3-year schools are using resources, time, and energy to meet the national standards for accreditation, these others are spending funds to promote an essentially retrograde movement. And, most serious of all, there has begun to be an organized effort outside of nursing to take from the nursing profession the right to determination of its standards for a segment of the schools of nursing offering basic preparation. Can any nurse fail to understand the significance of such a surrender of the prerogatives of her profession?

It is essential that all nurses respect the privilege of the profession to determine its own standards and goals. If serious incompatibilities arise, the more progressive and better educated may feel compelled to withdraw into separate organizations.

Fourteen years ago, when the earlier article on professional status was published, an intensive study of the structure of national nursing organizations was beginning. This study continued for several years with representatives of the several national societies meeting and considering reports of working committees and consultants. It was an instructive example of the serious-mindedness of the nursing profession in seeking to improve its working relationships.

When it had been agreed that the work of the profession could be accomplished by two organizations, these were set up, with appropriate functions assigned to each. In brief, the American Nurses' Association undertook "continuing improvement of professional practice, the economic and general welfare of nurses, and the health needs of the American public." The second organization, the National League for Nursing, now represents the interests of the National Organization for Public Health Nursing and the National League of Nursing Education. In NLN "all members of the health team, agencies supplying nursing service, and education, and lay members of the community, representing all races, creeds, and national origins act together to provide the best possible nursing services and to assure good nursing education."

The once separate organization for Negro graduate nurses has ceased to exist and now in all states of the Union, save one, all nurses may belong to the state constituent of the ANA. Practical nurses have been welcomed into the NLN. Structure continues to be studied, and there is a current proposal to consider consolidation of the present two organizations. These are all indications of a dynamic profession.

6. A profession attracts individuals of intellectual and personal qualities who exalt service above personal gain and who recognize their chosen occupation as a life work.

Certainly, nursing is continuing to attract individuals of intellectual and personal characteristics of a high order, and many of these are dedicated to nursing as a career of service. It has been frankly and straightforwardly admitted that marriage and a career in nursing may be considered divergent forces. Since World War II, however, women seem to have enhanced their ability to care for a family and also have a career. Moreover, nursing seems to have acquired a much more tolerant attitude toward the person who is both a nurse and a homemaker. Increasingly one finds the highly motivated intelligent person returning to school to pursue graduate study, even though she has one or several children, and then going back into increased responsibility in some nursing position. If all the nurses who have home responsibilities were removed from the nursing school faculties and hospital staffs, it would be impossible to staff either the schools or hospitals today.

One of the criticisms leveled at the graduate of collegiate programs by some who have presumably employed both the 3- and the 4-year product is that she isn't "as good a nurse" as the person who completes her preparation in a year's less time. This criticism should be examined thoroughly, for it seems highly probable that only a part of what is being expected of today's nurse is being tested in such an evaluation. If the allegation should have substance, it is a matter of great concern and must be righted, for few may be able to afford the luxury of the added year unless there is assurance that the product is prepared to go further in a shorter time after graduating.

7. A profession strives to compensate its practitioners by providing freedom of action, opportunity for continuous professional growth, and economic security.

In the 1945 article we said that the phrase, "strives to compensate," implies that professions can only imperfectly repay their practitioners by their service to society, and this continues to be true today. Society's appreciation of the services of the nurse seems to have grown, however. This is evidenced by the increasing prestige of the nurse in her participation in national and international groups of many disciplines, and in her role locally, too. It is evident also in the slowly improving economic gains of nurse groups, and in the numbers which by now are recognized in retirement and employee security programs of industry, education, and government.

A notable development which increases the opportunity for continuous professional growth is the larger number of scholarships and fellowships provided for use in nursing education. One much appreciated provision, for example, is administered by the National League for Nursing, largely through the generosity of the Commonwealth Fund. If a complete roster of contributors to the support of nursing students could be compiled, it would amaze the reader by its diversity and number. Some states are providing funds for the education of nurses; the Federal government has provided, in the past three years, a total running into the millions of dollars for fellowships for nurses.

An increasing number of today's nurses are qualifying for advanced education. Only a few years ago not enough well-prepared people could be found for the establishment of competent faculties in some of our largest universities! Also, as many and as valuable opportunities for professional growth are being provided in informal ways as in formal schooling. Best of all, nurses are entering more and more into the planning for their own professional growth.

In respect to economic security, significant progress should also be noted. Perhaps the most significant has been shown in the changed attitudes of nurses themselves toward undertaking their own economic security program and their acceptance of the principles of collective bargaining. Through the leadership of the ANA, the state nurses' associations have become more effective. Here, as in other parts of the program of the ANA, many individuals from other professions such as industrial relations experts, lawyers, sociologists, and economists, have been useful in assisting nurses to interpret their own needs. The strength of the position nurses have taken lies in part in their affirmation that the public shall not suffer, that nurses will not strike but will depend upon more constructive group action to adjust their problems with employers.

There may be those who doubt there is any place for bargaining in a real profession, but to such it can be said that the essence of democracy is in this principle, and while society has employers and employees, protection of the latter must be as well assured as privilege for the former. In times of rapid social and economic change, with living costs moving upward from month to month, it is especially necessary that those who are not self-employed have protection and also the freedom to discuss working conditions and pay for services with their employers and with each other.

One of the criteria for a profession is the existence of a professional association. It is the association that tends to set the standards for the profession and helps to enforce them. Some sociologists have argued that too rigid a stand by a professional association on licensing, educational qualifications, etc. tends to close the profession, slowing its growth and cutting it off from contact with new ideas. While this is a danger, nursing organizations have never been strong or powerful enough to make the nursing profession a closed one.

The nursing association has shown considerable change in function since its inception, as can be shown by the plans for the first nursing association. The first efforts to organize a nursing association in the United States were made at the International Congress of Charities, Correction and Philanthropy which was held in conjunction with the Chicago World's Fair in 1893. Though the ideas for a nurses' association were somewhat nebulous, they led to the Associated Alumnae groups (predecessor of the ANA) and the organization of superintendents (predecessor of the NLN).

11.
What a Nursing Association Should and Could Do (1893)

by Edith A. Draper

We have, as a profession, just emerged from infancy and attained our majority, it being twenty-one years since first an English woman introduced the system of training nurses in this country. A passing tribute to Sister Helen, the first superintendent of Bellevue, would not come amiss now, and could she see to what proportions her seedling has grown she would, I am convinced, feel amply repaid for her endeavors.

The plan so ably sketched some time ago, in our nursing periodical, through some misfortune has not matured. Whether the time was not pro-

From "Necessity of an American Nurses' Association," in Nursing the Sick. Isabel A. Hampton (ed.), Chicago, 1893. Reprinted under the sponsorship of the National League of Nursing Education. Copyright 1949. McGraw-Hill Book Company, pp. 149–53. Used by permission.

pitious, or a competent leader not forthcoming, or because energy and enthusiasm were lacking, or whatever the reason, to the majority of toilers for the sick in this broad land even the name of such an organization is utterly unknown.

We have gathered here from East and West, from far and near, actuated by the desire to take part in the World's Exhibition, this union of nations in one vast representation. It would be fitting to commemorate the time by adding our mite to the history of the Exhibition, and becoming an united organization, a body of women trained to be of unquestioned benefit to mankind and not lacking in love and sympathy for each other.

If I may urge the cause which appears to me so important a one for us, I would add that if we are ever to be ready for action surely now is the time. "There is a tide in the affairs of men which, taken at the flood, leads on to fortune." Surely the tide is high for us now and it were a thousand pities to allow so grand an opportunity to slip by. We represent a number of schools, our English friends are here to give us their experience and advice, the medical fraternity are ready to offer their support, and the way seems clear; our combined efforts will surely be crowned with success.

The difficulties to be encountered, one must truthfully admit, will be mainly of our own manufacture. What we need is energy of purpose, enthusiasm, a spirit of philanthropy more developed, and ambition to lift our profession to a height to which the eyes of the nation shall look up and not down. Nothing is more conducive to the ruination of a project than lukewarmness and a conservatism which does not look beyond individual benefits. These are our main hindrances, but not insurmountable ones, for though acknowledging these faults, we are aware of counterbalancing virtues and know that the day will come when America will be justly proud of this association of her countrywomen.

By a national association we mean a society with legal recognition, that every nurse who is a member of the same will be guaranteed for by the association and entitled to its benefits; and that we will be a recognized profession just as doctors are.

The objects to be attained would be schemes for professional and financial assistance, and, perhaps I should have put first, arrangements for conferences and lectures, that by meeting as frequently as possible we might gain a better knowledge of each other, which would result most undoubtedly in mutual appreciation, and consequently aid in the advancement of other schemes.

We have been accused, and with some justice, of envy, malice and all uncharitableness toward each other; schools of one system antagonistic to schools of another, and nurses of the larger cities and hospitals looking with contempt upon nurses trained in the smaller places. Upon this petty, narrow-minded state a quietus might be placed by the system of registering (for a standard of equality would be exacted), so that all members of the association would be considered equally competent as far as their technical knowledge went. To protect the public, the medical profession and ourselves, no better means have been suggested than this.

People may be spared, if they so desire, the imposition of the ignorant woman, who, not fit for anything else, is good enough for a nurse; from the so-called "natural nurse," who believes herself endowed from above with the necessary knowledge to undertake any case, no matter how critical, without wasting time on a preliminary training; from the rejected probationer, who endangers life with the infinitesimal scraps of information she has gleaned in a short stay in the hospital; and, lastly, from the woman who, expelled from her school for cause, pursues unchecked this means of livelihood.

To the many excellent women who have nursed successfully for years, without thorough training, it may seem an arbitrary measure that they should be excluded from the association; but if we are aiming at beneficial results to the many, the inconvenience to the few we may regret but cannot avoid.

I imagine we would all concur readily in deciding that the standard for membership be high; a certified diploma, at least two years training in a hospital, endorsements of work well done and testimonials of character above reproach, should be required.

As a means of discipline this association would prove a power. We might imitate the Society of Loyal Orangewomen, whose regulations state that a member will be fined or expelled who does not "behave as becometh an Orangewoman." An even more laudable undertaking would be the scheme for benefiting nurses in a financial way.

Notwithstanding the objections which have been raised on the score of patronage and the repugnance of the self-respecting toward anything savoring of charity, the assurance of material aid when overtaken by sickness, of a sufficiency to keep the wolf from the door when growing old and unable to discharge the arduous duties of a nurse any longer, would bring consolation and relief to many a weary worker.

In this country, though fairly well paid, nurses are not able to save to any great extent; whether the calls upon their slender means are too great, or possibly through sickness or their own improvidence, the fact cannot be controverted that pecuniary aid is not infrequently needed by members of our profession, and I imagine would be received without any loss of self-respect.

The Alumnae Associations furnish help by drawing upon members, and such help is not considered degrading: why should a larger and more far-reaching fund be so regarded?

If we can help others by lending our aid to this undertaking we must put aside all feelings which may tend to obstruct its advance. The endowment of beds for nurses in hospitals would meet with the approval of any nurse who has been ill in a boarding-house, and those of us who have not experienced this nightmare should, selfishly speaking, be most anxious to give our aid, as fortune may not always deal so kindly with us, and the vicissitudes which have overtaken others may in time overtake us.

Another and equally important aim would be the promotion of conferences and lectures as often as practicable. Those thoroughly interested in the work would find a way to attend occasional meetings, and each State association might send one or more representatives, so that in business matters all might have a voice; and through the medium of a publication, those unable to attend might keep up their interest. To advance we must unite! Otherwise, factions will arise and stagnation result. We know that nurses who have graduated ten or twelve years ago feel that they are not keeping pace with the advancement of medicine and science; that the recent graduate is oftentimes preferred before them, though in experience she may be a child. What better help can we give these nurses than the promotion of lectures, theoretical and practical, the encouragement of publications pertaining to our needs, and the free interchange of all the newest and best ideas?

Somewhere I have read that this plan is not feasible, and that we are sundered too far, geographically. We have immense territory to scatter over, it is true, but the difficulty does not seem to me insurmountable—rather an incentive to action.

I suppose the railways might be induced to give us excursion rates, annually. We are as deserving of consideration from them as the Christian Endeavor or any other society; and in the interim, lectures furnished by the Association and examinations held, something on the order of University Extension courses, would in each town or State be of inestimable value to those ambitious to be among the foremost in our calling. The opportunity to travel when annual meetings were held would be hailed with delight by every intelligent nurse and the appointment as delegate be regarded as an honor.

I have only touched lightly upon the many advantages to be obtained, and have not attempted any plan of organization. The subject is of vital interest to us all, and if I have succeeded in promoting its discussion my object has been attained.

The founders of the ANA were not quite sure what the functions of a professional organization should be, since these obviously vary with the type of organization. Some possible functions are set forth by the sociologist Robert K. Merton.

12.
The Functions of the Professional Association

by Robert K. Merton

The professional association is an organization of practitioners who judge one another as professionally competent and who have banded together to perform social functions which they cannot perform in their separate capacity as individuals. It is typically a voluntary association. The degree to which it is voluntary may, however, differ greatly from case to case. It may range from the extreme in which the option to join is small since the penalties of not belonging are great, as in the case of county medical societies, to the other extreme, in which the option is large since the penalties for not belonging are negligible, as in the case of the more than seventy-five national engineering societies.

Professional associations differ also in their structure. They may be closely controlled from a central office or may allow considerable autonomy to local branches of the association. I do not, however, intend to explore these variations of structure, important as they are, for it is not its structure which most significantly characterizes the professional society, but its functions.

The professional association *is* as the professional association *does*: its manifest and latent social functions, not the structure designed to put these functions into effect, are its social excuse for being. That is why we can largely neglect, in this short examination, the organizational structure of the association in order to center upon its functions.

Organizational Aims and Functions

Just as function must be distinguished from structure, so must function be distinguished from the stated objectives of the organization. Professional associations tend to be alike in putting into their statements of purpose a strong affirmation that they are designed, in the first instance, to work through

Reprinted, with permission, from *The American Journal of Nursing,* LVIII, 1958, 50–54.

their specialized competences for the welfare of the community in general and of their respective clienteles in particular. The American Medical Association announces as one of its principal aims the steady improvement of health care; the American Bar Association, the promotion of the administration of justice; the American Nurses' Association, the improvement of nursing care for all the people. And so, similarly, through the roster of the hundreds of professional associations, great and small, in this country.

What the association professes as its aims may coincide with what it actually does—but again, it may not. The statements of public purpose do provide guide lines for gauging the measures to be taken by the association. This is true for declarations designed not only to reach the general (that is, the professionally uninstructed) public but also, as everyone connected with such associations knows, to reach the membership of the organization itself. The declarations of high purpose are not merely window dressing, although they are in perpetual danger of becoming so. This is particularly the case when the profession confronts a crisis in which the interests of its members seemingly or actually conflict with the interests of the public.

Nevertheless, it would be too facile and often mistaken to assume that such statements of public purpose merely render lip service to social values. Even when they are being neglected in practice, they afford a potentiality of control over actions contemplated by the association and serve to bring these actions into line with the announced purpose.

Occasional or sometimes sustained departures of a professional association from its declared public purposes can result from the *multiple and not always easily reconcilable functions* of the association. For example, the association is committed to look out for the economic and social welfare of practitioners in the profession, for if the membership organization does not do so, who will? Again, it is typically dedicated also to the objective of raising the standards of professional education, for if the organized body of informed professionals does not take on this task, who else can? Yet sometimes objectives such as these, principled as they are, may collide, or many seem to collide, with the interests of the public. A profession with reason to suppose that its members are not receiving an income commensurate with their worth may press for a rise which many in the public will judge excessive. (This sort of thing helps form the image of the professions as a "conspiracy against the public," so energetically propagated by Bernard Shaw.) Or the association, on behalf of its apparently unimpeachable purpose of improving the competence of practitioners, may call for a great increase in public funds for advancing professional education. This capitalization of brain power may raise the cost of the (more effective) professional service. This, too, may not sit well with laymen who feel themselves twice penalized: once, by taxation and again, by higher fees for professional care. They can tell when the fiscal shoe pinches but they cannot so easily distinguish excellent professional care from good, and good from mediocre or inferior care.

Beyond these potential sources of conflict, there is the further possibility that a professional association may, for a time, come to be in the hands of those who conscientiously put the interests of the profession above all other interests, if only because they identify themselves so strongly with their profession that they can see the rest of the world only through the biased perspectives afforded by their professional spectacles.

It may be considered tactless to admit this possibility of a conflict of interest between a profession and the public, but it is unwise to deny it. Much as we should like it to be, we must not suppose that "all things work together for good." The social world is not inevitably a natural harmony of interests. At least in the short run, it is not the case that what is good for the profession of medicine or of law or of nursing is necessarily best for the community, and conversely. Only if these potential and actual conflicts are recognized and admitted, rather than put aside as an unpleasant embarrassment and systematically denied, can they be mitigated and worked out. The "irreconcilable" can be reconciled only if the sources of conflict are anticipated, continually appraised, and dealt with through that manner of equitable adjustment which man has proved, in his long history, he can occasionally achieve.

Every professional association faces the difficult task of trying to reach and to maintain a delicate balance between fulfilling its functions for the community and protecting its professional constituency from exploitation by the community. The not-too-distant days in which the nurse was rewarded for her dedication to high purpose by a dismally low income remind us that the balance can be lost at the expense of the professional group, just as numerous other instances remind us that it can be lost at the expense of the clientele.

This may be enough to suggest what I mean by saying that the public objectives affirmed by a professional association need not coincide with their actual functions. Now, if structure provides only the machinery for the performance of functions and if stated objectives provide only a guide to the selection of functions, what, then, are the basic functions which the professional association actually performs? Or, to substitute momentarily for the many-meaninged word "function," what do professional associations actually *do* and what are some of the ramified consequences of what they do?

Types of Social Functions

The professional association does so many things that, if we are to understand them, we must find a way of sorting them out into their several kinds. For this purpose, we can draw upon a way of thinking about the social functions of an organization which sociologists have found helpful. This involves designating the human units for which these activities are functional: individuals, subgroups, the organization, and the larger society. Some functions of the professional association primarily affect individual members of the profession (and indirectly their clientele); others have consequences primarily for the profession as a whole and for the association as its corporate expression; and still others primarily affect the larger social system in which individuals and organizations find themselves. This notation of kinds of multiple functions has the further merit of sensitizing us to the possibility that some activities of a professional association which are functional for one or more of these units can be dysfunctional for others—that is, can interfere with their adaptations—a possibility to which I have already referred.

Functions for Individual Practitioners

Perhaps the most pervasive and far-reaching function of the professional association for the individual practitioner consists in giving him social and moral support to help him perform his roles as a professional. The organization helps see to it that professional people need not cope with their professional problems alone. This supportive function does not require the organization to cater to their weaknesses; rather, it can serve to reinforce their strengths.

Particularly in the salaried professions, as distinct from the prevalently free-lance, fee-paid professions, the lone professional cannot effectively safeguard his social and economic welfare. There may be a considerable gap between the prevailing schedule of salaries and the schdule which, in all equity, should obtain. For generations, this has been notoriously true of the salaries of college professors. Whether through collective bargaining, which is still infrequent among professional associations, or through the less direct pressures of appeal to the public opinion, which is the characteristic though immediately less effective mode, the association works to reduce the extent of this gap between what is and what should be in the sphere of salaries.

The protective functions of the association for the individual practitioner are not limited to the narrowly economic matter of salaries. Others operate indirectly to improve his conditions of work. They are designed to enable him to do his professional job more effectively, to the further benefit of his clients. (The clientele, typically, shows no awareness of the benefits they derive from the work of the professional association.)

In the professions, as in all other forms of activity, sustained motivation is necessary for superior performance of roles. These motives to do well must be harnessed to the institutionalized system of rewards. This is one of the functions of associations, particularly of salaried professionals, which press for the provision of opportunities for advancement in accord with the growth of professional experience and competence of the practitioner.

The association works also to help prepare the practitioner for the more effective discharge of his professional roles. It acts on the philosophy that professional education is a lifelong process; establishes institutes to advance the education of the practitioner; protects both him and the public by working toward legally enforced standards of professional competence; and helps motivate practitioners to develop their skills and to extend their knowledge.

These and related functions can be summed up by observing that, in the professions, each practitioner *is* his brother's keeper. Each is expected to live up to or to exceed the acceptable standards of practice, and to see to it that others also do so. This means that the profession develops social and moral ties among its members who enter into a community of purpose. This cannot be accomplished under a system of *laissez-faire,* which can be freely translated, in this context, as a hands-off policy with each for himself and, in the ensuing disorder, let public indignation take the hindmost. It can be accomplished through an association of professional people which, through its solidarity of purpose, expresses a commitment to professional ideals and, through its solidarity of organization, polices both professionals and nonprofessionals to insure that conditions for living up to these ideals are provided.

This review, it may have been noted, has uniformly dealt with functions of the professional association for members of the profession rather than for members of the association only. This was not a lapse. It was meant to emphasize the important point that members of the profession who are not members of the association typically receive an unearned increment of social, moral, and economic gain from the work of their professional colleagues in the association. In the not inappropriate idiom, those who remain outside the organization are the "free-loaders": they do not pay their way, either in dues or in kind. True, the free-loaders in a profession often do not see themselves as such. They do not realize that they are nonpaying and nonparticipating beneficiaries of the sustained work done by those who make up the associations representing their profession. Yet they are in much the same condition as citizens who would avoid paying taxes and taking part in public service while benefiting from the taxes and activities of the rest who contribute to the commonwealth. It is a task confronting every professional association to convert the free-loader into the member, preferably an actively participating member, not only that he may do his share of the work which the organized profession needs to have done but also in order that his voice may be heard when the organization formulates its policies.

Functions for the Profession

We can now drop the first tier of functions—those for the individual practitioner—and proceed to the second, composed of functions for the profession as a whole. As I have suggested, although the same organizational activities tend to have both types of functions, some of these can be seen to operate primarily for individual practitioners and others primarily for the profession as a collectivity.

The foremost obligation of the association is to set rigorous standards for the profession and to help enforce them: standards for the quality of personnel to be recruited into the profession; standards for the training and education of the recruits; standards for professional practice; and standards for research designed to enlarge the knowledge on which the work of the profession rests. The association must be in the vanguard. The standards it sets must be more exacting than those with which the lay public might be content. After all, only the informed professionals can know the potentialities and not merely the current realities of professional practice. They are the custodians of the professional traditions of the past; through their constituted organizations, they must also try to anticipate the future and continually raise their sights.

To say that the professional association must be unendingly engaged in pressing for higher standards of personnel, education, research, and practice is to say that it is committed to dissatisfaction with the state of affairs in the profession as it is. At least in its charter of purposes, the professional association repudiates that final smugness which assumes that everything possible has already been attained. It is thereby committed to keeping members of the profession from resting easily on their oars, even if they should feel so inclined. They must be brought to see that today is tomorrow's history, that the motto of the Passavant Hospital holds for all the professions: "more than yesterday, less than tomorrow."

In this particular sense, the professional association is a kind of organizational gadfly, stinging the profession into new and more demanding formulations of purpose. It must therefore be prepared to become a target for hostile criticism by those members of the profession who find themselves or feel themselves disadvantaged by the continuing forward thrust toward raising the standards of the profession.

This is only another instance of the "non-contemporaneity of the contemporaneous," of the co-existence of generations. At any time in the history of a profession, its members are variously trained and variously competent, since they have entered the field at different times. The less highly trained, naturally enough, look with some displeasure, if not despair, at the rising standards of qualifications for professional practice. To cope with this familiar problem, organizations have invented the device of the "grand-father clause," which exempts current members from having to meet the newly instituted and more rigorous standards of the profession. Even so, there typically remains a residue of resistance and hostility toward the policy of heightening standards.

This is inherent in the process of growth of a profession and those who staff the professional association should know it. They should know that the life of officers in a forward-moving professional association is not a tranquil one. They should realize that an excess of tranquility may only register the growth of complacency in the profession and the decline of responsible criticism among its constituted representatives. They should sense that the quiet organizational life may only mean that the profession is not living up to the commitments which it, in effect, made when it accepted the monopoly of rights and immunities conferred on it by society. If the obligation to raise standards for the profession makes life difficult at times, it is only the price which the truly *professional* association must be prepared to pay.

Since the dynamic of every profession is provided by the growth of its specialized knowledge, the professional association has the further function of advancing research in its field, either directly through research agencies of the association or, more often, indirectly through help to other individuals and groups in the profession. It can provide a clearing house of professional knowledge; it can help make the research career a feasible and honorable one in the profession; it can work toward the expansion of opportunities for research. In this respect, the professional association has elements of the learned society just as in some of its protective functions for individual practitioners, it has elements, regulated by a professional ethic, of the trade union.

The function of facilitating research does not stand alone. If the results of research are not disseminated among the profession, they are inert, powerless to move the profession forward. The association therefore establishes professional journals devoted to the reporting and spreading of new knowledge as well as ancillary house-organ journals devoted to information on the changing role of the profession in society.

By working to raise the standards of personnel, education, practice, and research, the association best serves a latent function for the profession, a function not directly contemplated in these activities which have worth in their own right. To raise these standards tends to improve the social standing of the profession. It lays the groundwork for a deserved rise in social esteem. The rise of a profession in the eyes of the community is *not* merely the result of what is often described as "public relations," of persuading the public that the profession should be more highly regarded. As publicists know, the development of a "public relations" program is no adequate substitute for the reality to be reported.

The flow of authentic information to the public about what is actually taking place in the profession has as its principle role the narrowing or closing of the gap between these actual advances and the public understanding of what these mean for the quality of professional service. If the face which the profession presents to the public is more attractive than the reality, the temporary rise in social esteem will only be the prelude to a great fall. It is the task of the association to improve the effectiveness of the profession; the task of its department of public relations to see to it that the degree of improvement becomes widely known. The art of meiosis—that is, of sustained understatement— is the art appropriate to the public relations arm of a truly professional association.

Functions for the Society

The functions of the professional association for individual practitioners and for the profession are, in the main, conspicuous ones, readily identifiable by those who would look and see. But one of the association's principal functions for the society of which it is a part is far from evident; it has often gone wholly unnoticed. This is its function, as one of the great intermediate associations, to help prevent the atomization of society into a sand-heap of individuals, each intent on pursuing his own private interests. Such an atomized condition is a step toward totalitarianism, which consolidates power over these socially disconnected individuals into a single center. As one thoughtful observer of this process has described it for a case in which totalitarianism came to prevail:

The destruction of the independent labor unions in Nazi Germany was followed by the prohibition of independent economic organizations of every kind. It was not the fact of labor that was central; it was the social fact of *union*. All autonomous organizations were destroyed and made illegal: professions, service clubs, voluntary mutual aid groups, fraternal associations, even philatelist and musical societies. Such organizations were regarded, and correctly, by the totalitarian government as potential sources of future resistance, if only because in them people were brought together for purposes, however innocent, that did not reflect those of the central government. As organizations they interposed themselves between the people as a society and the people as the masses.*

In a word, the professional association helps furnish the social bonds through which society coheres. It provides unity in action, social cohesion even without contiguity. The association mediates between the practitioner and profession, on the one hand, and, on the other, their social environment, of which the most important parts are allied occupations and professions, the universities, the local community, and the government.

The association relates each profession to allied professions. These relations may be faulty—they often are—but they are less faulty than they would be were it not for the numerous organizational liaisons which typically develop. It should also be admitted, even though it be regarded as another tactless observation, that the association also seeks to validate the scope, not infrequently the expanding scope, of the jurisdiction of the profession and to safeguard it against the rival claims of neighboring professions and technical occupations.

This pressure toward expansion derives in part from advancement of professional knowledge. It often produces strains and stresses on the relationships between neighboring professions. This problem only underscores the importance of instituting and maintaining effective liaison between professions, for only if this is firmly established can the relationship bear the stresses which initially conflicting claims to jurisdiction impose upon it. Even so, it is wise to expect residual conflicts of interest between professions which remain unresolved. This is part of the costs of a pluralist society in which decisions about the appropriate division of professional work are not imposed from above. Without strong professional associations, the problem would probably be multiplied and intensified.

The many-sided relations of the profession to the government are also mediated through the professional association. To do more than mention this fact would be to enter upon a long and complex account. It is perhaps enough to refer to the continuing role of the association in formulating policies for legislative enactment and in monitoring proposed legislation which bears upon the work and goals of the profession.

In its relation with the varied groups which compose the social environment of the profession, the association must develop a sufficient consensus to be able to speak authentically and authoritatively on behalf of the profession. Were a profession such as nursing to be heard through some 400,000

* Nisbet, R. A. *The Quest for Community.* New York: Oxford University Press, 1953, pp. 202–203.

separate voices, with each professional nurse proclaiming her own views and sentiments, only cacophony could result. The association seeks to create a concert of purpose instead.

This presents the professional association with the great problem of achieving a flexible consensus of values and policies. It must not only appear to speak for the profession; it must stand on firm ground in doing so. Yet it must provide for dissent, even though it cannot allow dissent to result in noise. To accomplish this result—i.e., an adaptable consensus with full opportunity for responsible dissent—requires formidable feats of organization which cannot, of course, be adequately examined in this short paper. A few general observations may nevertheless be in order.

I begin with the tried, trite, and true proposition that the association must provide two-way avenues for communication: ideas, problems, prospects, experience, and objectives must come to the association from members of the profession, and these, having been examined by democratically elected representatives of the profession, must then go back to the constituency for review. Only the organization of local constituent groups can provide the forum in which issues can be threshed out before action on them is taken nationally.

The professional association, like other large-scale organizations committed to democratic procedure, is confronted with the enduring tempation to transform the avenues of communication into one-way streets, with information and decisions moving only from the top of the organization. Unless the structure provides for reciprocal communication, the association works through control from above, whatever its pretensions to the contrary.

A price must be paid for the two-way street; at times, an unconscionably heavy price. For to wait upon the informed comment, and not merely the reluctant assent, of a far-flung and varied constituency often slows up the rate of advancing the work of the profession. But though this is at times a heavy drag on progress, it is more often, I suspect, only a seeming one. For until the great majority of the profession are themselves persuaded of the merits of proposed changes, any changes which are instituted are apt to be nominal rather than genuine. Only the men and women doing the work of the profession can translate proposals for improvement into reality.

To be able to speak for the profession, the association must be representative of as many of the profession as possible. This means that the association must strive for what the sociologist describes as "completeness." By completeness is meant that all those eligible for membership actually are members. Of course, no professional association has achieved completeness and associations differ greatly in the extent to which they have approached it. After its first half-century, for example, the American Medical Association could count among its members only 9 percent of the 100,000 physicians then in practice; today, more than a century after its founding, somewhat more than two-thirds of physicians are enrolled.

Associations of about the same size may differ substantially in the degree to which they approximate completeness and, consequently, in the extent of the authority and influence they can exercise. That is why professional associations are in principle committed to the effort to enlarge their membership to include as large a proportion as possible of those eligible for membership. As spokesman for the profession, the association must strive to move ever closer to completeness, knowing that this will remain an asymptotic goal— one which is approached but never fully reached. In this way, the association can better serve the multiple functions which are both its obligation and its reward.

One of the most important aspects of a profession is autonomy, i.e., the control a profession has over its own standards and activities. Much of the energies of early nursing leaders as well as the activities of nursing organizations were directed at the passage of nurse practice acts to protect the title of registered nurse. As soon as nurses found themselves a legally defined occupation, they found they could also be held individually liable for their acts. The fact that nurses can be legally sued indicates that, in the eyes of the law, they are regarded as responsible professional persons. It might also indicate that nurses have enough income to make suing them seem worthwhile. Because of the growing number of lawsuits, the California Nurses Association in 1948 initiated a group liability insurance program for its members. Other associations followed suit. The legal basis of nursing and the recognition of nursing as profession is shown in the following article.

13.
The Law and the Nurse

by William C. Scott and Donald W. Smith

Most nurses are familiar with nurse practice acts. These acts generally prohibit the use of the term "Registered Nurse" or its equivalent by any person who has not met certain qualifications prescribed in the act. The act may go further and prohibit the practice of professional nursing by any person who has not qualified as a registered nurse. The belief of professional nurses, as expressed through their professional organizations, is that the states should require licensure of all who nurse for hire—whether they are professional or so-called practical nurses.

Violation of a nurse practice act is punishable by the penalty prescribed in the act—usually of a criminal rather than civil nature. Any person who poses as a registered nurse when she is not, or any nurse who goes beyond the bounds of nursing and practices medicine—as, for example, performing an appendectomy—without a license, would not be astonished to find herself subjected to fine or imprisonment—even if her little excursion into surgery does not produce fatal results.

Nurses are not, however, so clear as to the grounds and extent of their possible civil liabilities as distinct from criminal responsibilities.

Civil Liabilities

Any discussion of civil liabilities must begin by pointing out that there are two principal types of civil liability: (1) liability for breach of contract, and (2) liability for torts.

A breach of contract is a violation of some obligation to which a nurse or other person has agreed—either expressly, or, sometimes, by implication. An example is that of a nurse who buys an automobile on the installment plan and fails to meet the installments. Contractual obligations are sometimes referred to as *consensual* obligations, to indicate that they are created only with the *consent* (again, express or implied) of the person involved.

A tort, on the other hand, is a breach of a noncontractual obligation—one which the law imposes on a person regardless of his consent, such as the obligation to drive a motor car carefully, or not to commit assault and battery, or not to keep wild and ferocious animals on one's premises. Torts are often

From "The Nurse's Legal Problems." Reprinted, with permission, from *The American Journal of Nursing*, XLVIII April 1948, 243–45. The importance of this aspect of nursing is shown in a series of articles by Nathan Hershey in the *Journal* on the law and the nurse, started in 1962 and since continued.

subdivided into three classes: intentional, such as assault and battery; negligent, such as negligent injury to the person of another; and so-called "liability without fault," such as may be imposed in favor of an injured person upon the owner of an escaped lion, even though the escape was due to no negligence on the part of the animal's owner.

The form of civil liability in which nurses are most interested is tort liability, and particularly liability for negligent injuries to the persons of others, since that is the form of liability which nurses in their professional capacity are most likely to incur.

Many nurses do not appear to realize that, as a general rule, *all persons are liable for their own torts.* The truck driver who negligently runs down a pedestrian, the railroad engineer who negligently hits an automobile, is liable in damages for his injuries to the person or property of the aggrieved party. The confusion in the minds of many laymen is due to two facts: 1) If the wrongdoer was the "servant" (i.e., an employee under the control) of a "master" or employer and the tort occurred in the course of his employment, the employer is *also* liable for the tort (although the injured person cannot, of course recover twice for the same injury); and 2) since the employee usually has little, if any, money or property and the employer is usually comparatively responsible financially, the injured person customarily brings action against the employer and often forgets all about his rights against the employee.

We often have occasion to employ the services of persons whom the law does not consider to be our "servants," even in the broad sense in which the law uses that term. If, for instance, a patient employs a physician or a client employs an attorney, and the physician jabs a scalpel into a bystander or the attorney runs into a pedestrian while driving to court to represent the client, the patient or the client is not liable for the tort. The reason (according to the law) is that a physician or attorney is not under the conrol of the patient or client, and is therefore an "independent contractor"; and one who employs an independent contractor is usually not liable for the latter's *torts.* He may, however, be bound by the latter's *contracts.* For instance, a client who employs an attorney to represent him in litigation is usually bound by any stipulations or agreements into which the attorney may enter with counsel for the opposing side; and a customer who duly authorizes a real estate broker to buy or sell a house may be bound by the latter's contracts. Hence the importance of the distinction between torts and breaches of contract.

When, therefore, some states, such as New York, hold that a nurse employed by a hospital is an "independent contractor," they do not impose any new liability upon the nurse; but, by thus holding that a *hospital* is *not* liable for the nurse's negligence, they in effect compel a patient with a grievance to sue the nurse and thus, from a purely practical standpoint, increase the likelihood that the nurse, if proved guilty, will be required to respond in damages.

It may be well to point out that, at least in many states, the same act (or omission to act) may be both a tort and a breach of contract. For instance, a nurse might conceivably enter into an express, but more usually implied, agreement with a patient to nurse him carefully; if, then, she is negligent in counting sponges and the patient is injured, he might sue her for either the tort or the breach of contract. The contract, however, would probably not subject the hospital to any greater liability than before—not because it would have been impossible for the hospital to authorize the nurse to enter into the contract on its behalf, but merely because the court or jury would probably find, as a matter of fact, that the hospital had not done so and that the nurse had contracted solely on her own behalf.

What is Negligence?

Having established the basis of a nurse's liability for the consequences of her own negligence, we turn next to a consideration of the nature of negligence. Negligence, in civil cases, is usually defined as the failure to act as a reasonable man (or woman) would act under the circumstances. Whether a nurse or other person has been guilty of negligence is, therefore, a complicated question of fact; and, frequently, it is possible to make an equally convincing argument for either the affirmative or the negative of this question. However, in some instances more definite rules may come into play.

One of such rules is that the violation of a statutory prohibition which was designed for the protection of a class of the public will generally be considered negligence toward that class. If, for instance, a nurse practices medicine or a non-nurse poses as a registered nurse, there has been a violation of a statute designed to protect patients. The offender would, therefore, probably be held to have been negligent toward the patient, without the need of any further proof of negligence. Her unauthorized conduct would not, however, be any proof of negligence if she had run into a pedestrian on her way to the hospital, since the nurse practice acts and medical practice acts were not designed to protect the public from careless drivers of motor vehicles. On the other hand, the failure of a nurse to have a driver's license would, for obvious reasons, be highly relevant to the issue of negligent driving.

A second rule which may be invoked is that, even when there is no duty to act at all, there may be a duty not to act negligently. Thus, a nurse might pass by an injured man on the street without incurring any legal liability, leaving moral or professional considerations aside. If, however, the nurse volunteers to render aid and does so negligently, she may very well subject herself to liability for the consequences.

Nurses frequently are interested in questions relating to the boundary line between the practice of nursing and medicine. As already explained, a nurse who crosses the boundary line is in an extremely vulnerable legal position, especially if any unfortunate consequences to the patient result; and even if no civil liability results, she is still guilty of a violation of the medical practice act. There is frequently, however, grave doubt as to whether she has crossed this sometimes hazy boundary. The practice acts usually define the professions of medicine and nursing in broad and general terms, which may be of little assistance in deciding to which profession a particular function legally belongs. When the opinion of both professions is unanimous that a particular duty is properly within the field of nursing, a nurse ordinarily has little occasion to fear either criminal or civil prosecution, not only because of the unlikelihood of prosecution for the performance of such a duty (unless negligently performed), but also because of the weight which courts or juries would be inclined to give to professional opinion (although such opinion would not necessarily be conclusive). When, however, professional opinion is not unanimous or the medical and nursing professions disagree upon the allocation of a function, the nurse may be in the position of performing the function at her peril.

It will be possible within the scope of this article to indicate only briefly some of the methods which the nursing profession might use to settle disputed jurisdictional questions (if one may borrow the term from the field of industrial relations). Since in the United States the medical and nursing professions are regulated by the states rather than by the federal government, the steps indicated (particularly the first and third) would probably be most feasible on a state-wide rather than nation-wide basis. The appropriate agency to consider and carry out such steps would, therefore, be the state nurses' association or other state professional nurses' organization most concerned with the particular matter involved.

The first step to consider is the possibility of obtaining an authoritative written opinion from the highest state officer concerned with the enforcement of the medical and nurse practice acts. Usually this officer is the state attorney general. In some states, the attorney general may follow a policy of rendering formal opinions only upon the request of a department of the state government. In such case, resort may sometimes be had to obtaining an "informal" written opinion. If this cannot be done, the head of a state hospital, the state board of nurse examiners, or some similar authority may be prevailed upon to request the attorney general for his opinion and to make it generally available to the profession in states where such opinions are not regularly published. The opinion of an attorney general, while not binding on a court, is usually given great weight, and is frequently the best available prediction as to how a court would decide the question.

Secondly, the nursing profession should consider the possibility of meeting with representatives of the medical profession for the purpose of settling disputed questions by agreement. Such agreements between the organizations of the two professions would lead to the unanimity of professional opinion previously discussed as advantageous to the nurse. If both professions agreed that a given task was properly a part of nursing, the nurse would have less worry in performing it. If, on the other hand, both professions agreed that only a physician could properly perform it, she would have fewer qualms in protesting if a physician or hospital directed her to perform the task. Agreements between organizations representing different professions would not constitute an innovation; there are precedents in other professions if the nurses and physicians wish to follow them.

Finally, in appropriate cases, nurses might endeavor to obtain the passage of a clarifying amendment to their state nurse or medical practice acts. Where the matter is not merely doubtful but also controversial, it would unquestionably be advantageous first to reach agreement with the medical profession, since the matter would thus be taken out of the realm of controversy and the two professions could then present a united front to the legislators. If, however, such agreement could not be reached, the nursing profession might be obliged to take its case directly to the legislature—if only to "smoke out" the real desires of their medical colleagues. It has been reported, for example, that physicians occasionally declare certain duties to be the exclusive prerogative of the medical profession and at other times insist on ordering nurses to perform such duties. Obviously, in such circumstances, the physicians should not be permitted to have it both ways; and it may be doubted, if the matter were brought to their attention, whether they would wish to do so. Certainly, there would appear to be every reason at the present time to hope that any doubtful questions can be settled by amicable agreement between the professions.

One final word of caution. Acts and omissions to act do not exist in a vacuum. An act which a nurse should not perform on her own responsibility may be quite proper when performed under the immediate supervision of a physician. The value of obedience and discipline is too great to require the nurse constantly to question the propriety of the orders given her. Except under unusual circumstances, a nurse should be able to consult her state nurses' association and obtain authoritative advice before she objects the next time she is asked to perform a doubtful function. But the state nurses' association will be unable to give her such authoritative advice so long as the law itself is unclear and so long as the matter is a subject of professional controversy. While, therefore, in general, it is advantageous to phrase practice acts in broad language rather than to attempt to enumerate all the multifarious duties of a profession,—to say nothing of the duties which do *not* belong to a profession,—occasions may arise when, in simple justice to the perplexed practitioners of the profession, it is better to make an exception and to state specifically in the statutory law that a particular duty is or is not one of the proper functions of a profession.

One final mark of a profession is the existence of a rigorous professional code and standards. Nursing was rather late in establishing such a code, and one of the reasons for adopting the code was to meet the definition of a profession. The code, first adopted by the ANA in 1950, was revised in 1960. It states:

Professional status in nursing is maintained and enriched by the willingness of the individual practitioner to accept and fulfill obligations to society, co-workers, and the profession of nursing.

The following statements constitute a guide for each individual nurse in fulfilling these obligations.

1. The fundamental responsibility of the nurse is to conserve life, to alleviate suffering, and to promote health.

2. The nurse provides services based on human need, with respect for human dignity, unrestricted by considerations of nationality, race, creed, color or status.

3. The nurse does not use professional knowledge and skill in any enterprise detrimental to the public good.

4. The nurse respects and holds in confidence all information of a confidential nature obtained in the course of nursing work unless required by law to divulge it.

5. The nurse as a citizen understands and upholds the laws and performs the duties of citizenship; as a professional person the nurse has particular responsibility to work with other citizens and health professions in promoting efforts to meet health needs of the public.

6. The nurse has responsibility for membership and participation in the nurses' professional organization.

7. The nurse participates responsibly in defining and upholding standards of professional practice and education.

8. The nurse maintains professional competence and demonstrates concern for the competence of other members of the nursing profession.

9. The nurse assumes responsibility for individual professional actions and

judgment, both in dependent and independent nursing functions, and knows and upholds the laws which affect the practice of nursing.

10. The nurse, acting through the professional organization, participates responsibly in establishing terms and conditions of employment.

11. The nurse has the responsibility to participate in study of and action on matters of legislation affecting nurses and nursing service to the public.

12. The nurse adheres to standards of personal ethics which reflect credit upon the profession.

13. The nurse may contribute to research in relation to a commercial product or service, but does not lend professional status to advertising, promotion, or sales.

14. Nurses, or groups of nurses, who advertise professional services, do so in conformity with the dignity of the nursing profession.

15. The nurse has an obligation to protect the public by not delegating to a person less qualified any service which requires the professional competence of a nurse.

16. The nurse works harmoniously with, and sustains confidence in nursing associates, the physician, and other members of the health team.

17. The nurse refuses to participate in unethical procedures and assumes the responsibility to expose incompetence or unethical conduct in others to the appropriate authority.

Nursing has adopted a code of ethics, the ANA is an organization that meets most of the minimal requirements for a professional association, and nurses themselves have taken some steps towards claiming recognition as professional persons. The question is whether they want to go all the way or rather remain as they are today.

III THE NURSING ROLE

The role of the nurse, particularly that of the hospital nurse, has gone through a series of changes in recent years. Instead of offering a single level of patient care, nursing service in the modern hospital is made up of a complex system of practitioners, including nurses' aides, licensed practical nurses, registered nurses with various specialties, and several levels of nursing administrators. Registered nurses have viewed this growing complexity with a certain amount of ambivalence. Investigations of student attitudes have shown that most nursing students come into nursing because of a desire to help people or to give direct patient care. Yet the change of roles has left the direct patient care to practical nurses or nurses aides, while the registered nurse increasingly gives only the more involved and highly technical kinds of nursing care and coordinates the work of the various paramedical practitioners. This has led some observers to argue that nursing care has become so fragmented that the patient is left without a feeling of continuity of care and without the emotional support that the general duty nurse used to give. Some commentators feel that since direct patient care is the essence of nursing, the professional nurse rather than other nursing practitioners should have this role. Other observers claim that the role differentiation that has taken place was necessary or at least inevitable, and suggest that "team" nursing is a good way to organize the various hospital workers.

The role separation in nursing, however, is not new, but dates from the time of Florence Nightingale. When the Nightingale nurses first appeared, they were conceived of as "lady" nurses, a group far removed from nurses of the past who lacked the education and training that Miss Nightingale felt was necessary to give adequate nursing care. Thus from the beginning of modern nursing, there have been at least two competing groups of nurses. Education programs of the early twentieth century created a further division since hospitals were almost entirely run with student nurses, while the registered nurse either served as a supervisory teacher or went on the registry.

95

The nurse's view of her own role has also changed. This is evident from an examination of the views of some of the American pioneer nurses. Lavinia L. Dock, feminist, agitator for popular reform, and early socialist, was in favor of a rigidly prescribed structure within the nursing school, quite different from the beliefs she held towards events outside the hospital.

14.
Nurses Should Be Obedient

by Lavinia L. Dock

Absolute and unquestioning obedience must be the foundation of the nurse's work, and to this end complete subordination of the individual to the work as a whole is as necessary for her as for the soldier. This can only be attained by a systematic grading of rank, a clear, definite chain of responsibility, and one sole source of authority, transmitted in a straight line, not scattered about through boards and committees, but concentrated in the head of the school as their representative and delegate. They cannot represent themselves; they cannot do her work, nor exert her influence. She must do this herself, and there is no danger of making her an autocrat if they will consistently maintain their own just and true position, that of wise advisers, or judges if need be. Most unsound is the policy of the hospital which habitually interferes in the affairs of the school; and the most undignified expression of weakness of this kind is that which gathers up from women in training, who have not yet proved their merit, opinions, information, or complaints upon school or hospital matters.

It may be claimed that if the military idea is the basis of the school, the members of the medical profession being undoubtedly the superior officers, should properly control the school throughout its entire course, and even in its internal management, and that the whole subject of the teaching, training and discipline of nurses should be at the discretion of medicine. This might hold good except for one simple yet radical point of difference. The private soldier in the ranks and the officer in command have the same pro-

From "The Relation of Training Schools to Hospitals," a paper given before the International Congress of Charities, Correction, and Philanthropy at the Chicago World's Fair in 1893. It was published in *Nursing the Sick,* Isabel A. Hampton (ed.), Chicago, 1893 and reprinted under the sponsorship of the National League of Nursing Education, New York: McGraw-Hill Book Company, 1949, pp. 12–24. (Extract).

fession. The officer is also a soldier and knows every detail of the common soldier's work and life. The nurse and the physician have different professions. The doctor is not a nurse, and only now and then is one found who fairly comprehends the actual matter-of-fact realities of the training school. On this fundamental difference rests the claim of the school to be ruled, as an educative and disciplinary body, by those of its own origin. For another reason the separation of the medical power from training school affairs should be rigidly enforced, and that is the destructive effect of personal influence on the idea of duty. In hospitals about us may be seen the results of giving the hospital staff any practical hold over the school. What, for instance, is the consequence of allowing young internes to choose their own undergraduate head-nurses? The standard of the work is at once lowered by the introduction of the personal element. The pupil nurses are exposed to the temptation of seeking the favor of individuals. Partisan cliques invariably form, whose self-interest may be directly opposed to the best interests of the hospital and its nursing work; and promotion on a true merit-basis is utterly and at once impossible. In the struggle against influences of this kind the school is likely to be unjustly condemned by the hospital as troublesome. Arbitrary, insubordinate, its head as the natural enemy of the medical staff; a false position into which, by unfairness and jealousy, she is sometimes ungenerously forced.

On one field only does the school properly come under the command of the medical profession, and that is in the direct care of the sick. Here indeed the command is absolute. The whole purpose of the school centers around this point, and the pride of the well-drilled nurse is to make this service perfect.

Now for the first time in the history of medical science can its orders be carried out faithfully, fully, and at all hours. The uselessness of expecting such obedience from even intelligent persons who have not been trained is well illustrated by the remark of a lady of position and education, concerning the orders given her by the physician for her child's diet. "I shall do just half of what the doctor said," she observed, "as I always make a discount for each doctor's own particular fad."

From the beginning of organized nursing, there were a great many people who served as nurses who were not registered nurses. The practical nurse or nurse attendant existed before the trained nurse and continued to exist alongside of the developing professional nurse. Since most nursing before World War II was private duty nursing, graduate nurses often competed with the untrained practitioners for a job. It was as an attempt to find a solution to this problem, yet maintain educational standards, that Josephine Goldmark and the Committee for the Study of Nursing Education urged that there be at least two levels of trained nursing practitioners.

15.
The Need For an Auxiliary Nursing Service

by Josephine Goldmark
and the Committee for the Study of Nursing Education

When we find that certain private physicians, like the public health administrators, demand nurses of a higher quality than those now in the field, while others desire merely "hands for the physician" with a minimum of education below the present standard, it seems probable that there is reason on both sides and that the apparent conflict is due to a difference in the objectives to be met. For the care of acute and serious illness and for public health work it seems certain that we need high natural qualifications and sound technical education; for the care of mild and chronic illness and convalescence it may well be that a different type of capacity and training may be necessary.

It seems clear to the Committee, however, that, if two types of nursing service are desirable, the distinction should be drawn, not on economic grounds, but according to the type of illness involved. We are even somewhat doubtful as to the possibility of attaining very substantial economies by the introduction of a subsidiary type of private duty nurse. Our survey of the situation does not indicate that the income of the private duty nurse is at present generally an exorbitant one, when we take into account the amount of unemployment,—amounting in a typical group of 118 nurses to a week each month during the busy winter season. If this factor be allowed for, the

From *Nursing and Nursing Education in the United States.* New York: The Macmillan Company, 1923, pp. 14–16.

margin between the average annual income of the private duty nurse
and that of the domestic servant is not so great as to permit of the existence
of an intermediate grade on a salary level very much below that of the
present registered nurse. The solution of the economic problem which confronts the family of low income must probably be sought along the lines
of cost distribution through some form of community organization, or along
the lines of group insurance such as that being experimentally tested in New
York City.

In any event, a pneumonia case, a diphtheria case, a grave cardiac case
will require the highest grade of nursing obtainable, whether it occurs in a
palace or a hovel. It is the mild and chronic and convalescent case which
offers a field for the partially trained worker, and the exact extent of this
field has never yet been fully surveyed. In our own study we have secured careful estimates from 118 graduate nurses which indicate that during a period
of 3 months one quarter of their time was spent on cases which could have
been cared for by an attendant of the partially trained type. A somewhat
similar estimate was obtained from 48 practising physicians, 21 believing that
trained nurses were unnecessarily employed for less than a quarter of their
cases, 17 placing the figure between half and three-quarters, and 10 at over
three-quarters.

In considering the problem of subsidiary nursing service it must be remembered that we are dealing with no new development. Of the 300,000 male
and female nurses in the United States in 1920, slightly more than half were
of grades below the standard of the graduate nurse. The "practical nurse,"
the "trained attendant," is an existing fact; and in the opinion of a large group
of the medical profession who utilize her services she fills a real place in
the complex problem of caring for the sick.

If we include with the trained and registered nurses (149,128) the student nurses in hospitals (54,953) and to these add the number of attendants
and practical nurses (151,996), as constituting the entire body of persons occupied in caring for the sick, we have altogether one nurse, trained or untrained, to every 294 well persons. This would seem to give an adequate
supply if numbers alone are considered, provided a proper distribution could
be secured.

On the other hand the danger in the existence of a loosely defined and un-
regulated group of partially trained workers, in the same field as a more
highly educated type, constitutes a real and a serious complication. The
nursing profession has discharged a fundamental duty to the public in stimu-
lating the development of registration laws which define and delimit the
practice of that profession, and protect the community against fraud and
exploitation by those who collect fees and assume responsibilities to which

their qualifications do not entitle them. In addition to the registration of the trained nurse it is essential that the lower grade of nursing service should also be defined and registered; and the states of New York, Missouri, California, Michigan, and Maryland have taken definite steps in enacting legislation toward this end. The name to be selected for the subsidiary group is a difficult problem. As is so often the case the root of disagreement lies largely in nomenclature. The title "attendant," embodied in three of the laws mentioned above, is distasteful to those who bear it and tends to discourage the enlistment of those who may desire to enter this field. On the other hand the term "practical nurse" assumes a most unfortunate antithesis between education and practice; and the splendid professional and public service rendered by "the nurse" in war and in peace, entitles her to the protection of her existing professional status. We are inclined to believe that the term "nursing aide" or "nursing attendant" best meets the need for clear differentiation, while providing the subsidiary worker with a suitable name.

With two distinct grades of service available, the individual physician would be responsible for the choice of a trained nurse or a nursing attendant or nursing aide in a given instance. The public can be safeguarded in these matters only by state legislation providing for licensing of nursing registries and requiring explicit statement as to the license qualifications of each nurse or nursing aide furnished. We believe that by this means the maximum increase of nursing service possible under existing economic conditions could be attained; and we would therefore recommend that steps should be taken through state legislation for the definition and licensure of a subsidiary grade of nursing service, the subsidiary type of worker to serve under practising physicians in the care of mild and chronic illness, and convalescence, and possibly to assist under the direction of the trained nurse in certain phases of hospital and visiting nursing.

Ideas similar to those of Josephine Goldmark, namely, that there be two levels of nursing practitioners, had also been expressed by Dr. Charles Mayo, one of the famed founders of the Mayo Brothers Clinic in Rochester, Minn. In a widely publicized interview with Genevieve Parkhurst, ("Wanted— 100,000 Girls for Sub-Nurses," *Pictorial Review,* October, 1921, 82), Dr. Mayo had suggested that 100,000 country girls be trained two years to act as "sub-nurses" because, "The educational standards for registration of nurses set down by the nursing boards of the various states have gone beyond all reason. . . . The laws of most states demand high school pre-education and three years of training for the registered nurse; the only way to circumvent them is by training sub-nurses or nursing aids who will accept smaller pay, whose demands will not be so exacting, and who will be proficient enough to take hold of almost any case presented them." As a result of Mayo's remarks, the mere suggestion of training second level nursing personnel was regarded as an attack on the basic foundation of nursing. (This at least is the impression given by an editorial in the *American Journal of Nursing XX* November, 1921, 73.)

Strengthening the nurses' refusal to consider a division of the nursing role was the growing unemployment of graduate nurses. A more or less official reaction to any such suggestion is found in the Report of the Committee on the Grading of Nursing Schools, commonly known as the Burgess Report.

16.
There Is No Need for a Short Course Nurse

by May Ayres Burgess

Physicians agree that from the point of view of the patient, the private duty nurse costs too much. They are considerably more impressed with this difficulty, apparently, than even the patients themselves; although, of course, the patient questionnaires frequently deal with the same problem. The medical profession has for several years been keenly concerned with the cost of nursing care and, as a result, many suggestions have been made for lower-

From *Nurses, Patients and Pocketbooks.* New York: The Committee on the Grading of Nursing Schools, New York: 1928, pp. 463–471. (Extract).

ing the cost and so bringing nursing within the reach of the average patient. Perhaps the commonest suggestion, and one which has been made frequently by physicians in this study, has been that of trying to secure a "short course" or "basic" nurse.

The testimony has been rather surprisingly uniform and emphatic in its criticism of the so-called "practical" nurse. Contrary to the impression held by many nurses, it is not true that physicians generally are employing practical nurses for their own patients. Most physicians not only are actually employing R.N.'s but definitely prefer R.N.'s. Their experience with practical nurses while occasionally happy, is, for the most part, so extremely unsatisfactory that, as one physician said, "One comes to feel that all so-called 'practical' nurses ought to be deported!"

The comments on the undergraduate nurse are in some cases even more vitriolic than those relating to the frankly untrained. The criticisms for both groups may be summarized under the four words: *Ignorant, Incompetent, Uncooperative, Costly.*

Many cases have been reported to the Grading Committee of practical nurses who are charging more than the standard price for R.N. service. For the entire study the reports show that the typical practical nurse costs only $1 a day less than the typical R.N. Physicians are almost uniform in their protest against the types of practical nurses usually available and against their excessively high charges.

It is not wholly easy to understand why rather a large number of physicians who have had experience with the practical nurse and who are frank in their condemnation of her methods seem to feel that a new group of semi-trained workers would somehow avoid the undesirable characteristics of which they complain in the present supply.

When the physicians describe the "basic" nurse, the plan seems to be about as follows:

1. They would like to secure girls of fine breeding with reasonably good minds and—this is especially emphasized—a large amount of tact.

2. The girl should have had at least one or two years of high school.

3. She should be sent to a hospital which is willing to take her for a 12 or 18 months course.

4. After finishing the course, she should concentrate on private duty in the home.

5. She should specialize in 24 hour service.

6. She should be willing and competent to handle the more important parts of the house work.

7. She should never charge more than $25 a week.

The specifications in different communications vary, of course. One physician suggested that these girls be recruited from newly arrived immigrants, another suggested that the graduates of these courses should never be allowed to charge more than $15 a week, but the general outline seems to run about as listed above.

After reading some of the reports of physicians and nurses, a member of the Grading Committee remarked that apparently the chief difficulty in private duty was because, side by side with the gentlewomen whom we think of as nurses, servant girls *had* been allowed to enter the profession. "The mercenary spirit," "the negligence while on duty," "the impudence," "the overbearing attitude towards servants," and the various other characteristics of which frequent complaint has been made, are to any employer of domestic labor unfortunately all too familiar.

It is not believed that the difficulty in private duty is that most nurses are too well-bred or too well educated. There is, of course, the occasional nurse from a good family and with a high school or college education who has an unpleasant personality, but one gains the definite impression that most of the serious criticisms directed at private duty service are based upon the experience of patients and physicians with the servant girl element in the profession, and not with the rank and file.

In talking with hospital administrators it has seemed increasingly clear that very few hospitals are anxious to run short courses. The hospital loses money on the completely untrained student. It is only after a few weeks and sometimes after several months that the new student becomes sufficiently familiar with hospital routine so that she is an asset and not a liability. It seems probable that very few hospitals would be cordial to the proposition that they should carry the brunt of introducing students into hospital technique and then, at the very time when they are beginning to pay their way, should let them go and take on a new group of untrained young women. It is the third year of the student service which makes the hospital want to run a training school, not the first year.

One is inclined to believe that hospitals do not generally look with favor upon establishing 12 month or 18 month courses. It would also seem that unless entrance requirements in regular nursing schools are almost uniformly raised to high school graduation (and while this is probably desirable, it is undoubtedly some years in the future), comparatively few young women can be persuaded to enter the short term courses.

Evidence has already been presented in this report to indicate that students are definitely attracted by high entrance requirements and not by low ones. It does not, therefore, seem probable that any great increase in cheap labor would be secured by a campaign for short term courses for practical nurses.

There is reason to doubt whether the product would be satisfactory. Apparently there is general agreement that at least two years of eight hours a day of service on the floor are necessary in order to prepare graduate nurses for bedside care. The common criticism of graduate nurses is that even with these long hours of practical bedside experience, they are inadequately grounded in bedside technique. It would seem logical to suppose that the student who has had half or a third of the amount of bedside experience would prove unsatisfactory to the physician's needs.

There seems no reason to assume that the short term nurse would charge any less than the present practical nurse. One is inclined to believe that the fact that hospitals were sponsoring such graduates would be used by them as an argument for charging as much or more than the registered nurse now charges.

Finally, one would question whether there is any good reason for seeking to increase the number of semi-trained, relatively incompetent, inadequately educated young women in a field which is already oversupplied with material of that sort. It is an unfortunate fact that many low grade women have been admitted to the nursing professions and are actually registered and practising. The problem would seem to be, "How can such women who are already in the profession be placed under some form of guidance so that they can be an asset and not a danger to the community?" There seems no strong argument in favor of increasing this social burden.

The problem of the cost of nursing care is an extremely serious one. To the average patient with a long illness the expense is often excessive. It would not seem, however, that the solution is to keep on with present methods of distribution by attempting to lower the standard of living for nurses. The problem must be squarely faced and better methods of distribution somehow devised so that the cost of nursing care can be lowered to the patient while the standard of living for the individual nurse can accord with that of other professional women. There must be possible solutions for this problem which will work out to the mutual satisfaction of the nurse, the patient, and the physician.

This discussion can be summarized as follows:

1. Physicians are even more emphatic than patients in stating that the private duty nurse costs too much. Patients also, however, often stress this point.

2. Physicians and patients are agreed in their dislike for most so-called practical and undergraduate nurses. They ordinarily avoid them when they can.

3. Some physicians seem to feel that a new type of practical, semi-trained, or short course nurse might be produced who would solve the cost problem, while avoiding the defects of present practicals and undergraduates.

4. The picture they draw seems impracticable. It calls either for women above the servant level to accept, without special reason, conditions which servants will not tolerate; or for women at or below the servant level voluntarily to forego opportunities for personal advancement.

5. Some solution must be found for the excessive cost of nursing service. It is believed that this solution will come not through adding more incompetents to an already overcrowded field, but rather through devising new methods of distribution, so that the cost of nursing care can be lowered for the patient, while at the same time the standard of living for the individual nurse can be maintained at a reasonably adequate level.

World War II marked the emergence of the hospital as the chief employer of nurses. The importance of the hospital grew with changes in diagnostic technique, the development of medical insurance, and new kinds of medical treatment. As a result, the hospitals more than before served patients from middle and upper income groups, people who would have relied on home care in the past. Private duty nursing rapidly declined in importance. At the same time the demands of the Armed Forces for nurses tended to create a shortage of nurses; one nurse in four was in the service. The hospital, by its complexity, encouraged a division of labor among nurses, a specialization encouraged also by the Armed Forces which supplemented their nursing staffs with medical technicians. To alleviate the nursing shortage, many hospitals, both military and civilian, recruited nurses' aids. The Red Cross, in cooperation with the Office of Civilian Defense was a leader in this effort, although there was considerable opposition from the nurses themselves. Many of these aides who started as volunteers became paid employees after a brief time. When the war ended it was obvious that the shortage of nurses was not a temporary wartime phenomenon but a lasting one. The question then became one of how best to use another level of worker within the hospital situation. The national nursing organizations initiated several studies, the most influential of which was the report by Esther Lucile Brown. Dr. Brown advocated a differentiation of nursing on the basis of function, and it was her ideas on the role of the nurse that have dominated many of the recent developments in nursing.

17.
The Need For a Differentiation of Nursing Service

by Esther Lucile Brown

What then is a possible solution of this very difficult problem of obtaining a supply of nursing care that is quantitatively and qualitatively sufficient? Along with many other persons, we believe that the answer is inherent in the questions: What kinds of *nursing functions* need to be performed? Can persons be found and prepared to fulfill these *functions* effectively, whether they be graduate nurses or not?

One basic error, common to some other professions as well, has been primarily responsible, we believe, for the difficulties currently encountered. Emphasis has been centered upon "the nurse," or at best "nurses." The term as employed by the nursing profession and the laity responsible for making policy, moreover, has almost always meant the graduate nurse, the R.N., or the trained nurse as she used to be called. The fact that less economically and educationally advantaged persons often visualized a practical nurse when the term "nurse" was used has had little influence on the higher levels of thought and action. Had its influence been larger, at least the frame of reference might have been profitably broadened.

Emphasis, we are convinced, should have been placed squarely on *nursing,* and on *nursing functions* conceived of in their evolutionary and dynamic, not static, aspects. So long as attention is centered on the graduate nurse, no other avenue is open except that of the present frantic and probably futile effort to recruit more prospective R.N.'s. Even appreciably better educational preparation is likely to be denied them, so insistent will the demand for nursing service continue to be. Once emphasis is shifted to *nursing,* however, several roads seem to point to potentially larger supplies of service and to possibly increased efficiency both on the nonprofessional and the professional levels.

Pressure of circumstances has been leading steadily toward those roads. Unfortunately the experience gained has not been sufficiently examined, assimilated, and fashioned into a philosophy for planned future action. For a long time two systems of nursing care have existed side by side. So fixedly, however, have eyes been focused on one of those systems—that of graduate nurses—that the other, if recognized at all, has merely received the designation of "auxiliary." Only recently and in a relatively small number of places have any profound efforts been made to fuse members of these two systems into *coordinated teams* in which each person, according to background, training, and experience, performs certain functions essential to total nursing care.

From *Nursing for the Future.* New York: Russell Sage Foundation, 1948, pp. 57–72.

The System of Nongraduate Nursing Service

Practical nurses have probably existed for as long as persons have been hired to tend the sick. That they have often been highly incompetent because of lack of selection, training, and supervision, does not nullify the importance of the role that they have played in the home and that they can be trained to play far more effectively.

Because graduate nurses or large funds are not available, attendants have provided the predominant part of the bedside care given in hospitals for the mentally ill, and for chronic, convalescent, and tuberculous patients. They even constitute the major part of the nursing provided the acutely ill in some large municipal and county general hospitals. Their technical skill and understanding of patients have ranged from extreme limitation to remarkable ability. However that may be, the important fact here is that they have been and are now the only considerable source for staffing groups of institutions that probably contain over one-half of all the hospital beds in the United States.

The orderly, moreover, has had a long career in the general as well as the specialized hospital, particularly in the care of men patients. That he, too, has often been inefficient and has performed duties for which he was unprepared without adequate supervision is no denial of the essential place he has filled. Within a well-coordinated team, with better in-service training, his efficiency could be greatly increased.

The practical nurse, the attendant, and the orderly represent the large core of the system of assistant nursing service. The past two decades, however, have seen the ranks of that system markedly increased and broadened. Ward maids began to appear in voluntary hospitals when student and graduate nurses were no longer willing to do so much maid service, and when the hospital discovered the economy in employing them for such work. Although they do not directly provide nursing care, they have freed large segments of the time of nurses to give that care. They are an indispensable unit of the personnel of every ward. Attendants gradually made their entrance into voluntary hospitals before the outbreak of the recent war. Routine duties such as the making of empty beds, the carrying of trays, and the doing of simple tasks for patients were assigned to them. They also provided an important instrumentality in releasing nurses to give medications, treatments, and other more truly nursing care.

Then came Pearl Harbor and the drastic stringency of subsequent years. In order to keep hospitals in operation a wide and often strangely assorted variety of personnel had to be employed. Receptionists, errand boys, ward secretaries, voluntary workers in and out of uniform, and helpers of many designations appeared in bewildering numbers. Assistant workers of the attendant type were sought far and wide; much less consideration than formerly was given to their national origin, marital status, or color of skin. Although the major field of the practical nurse had formerly been private practice in the home care of the sick, every obtainable person so trained was pressed into hospital service,* or to a small degree into the hourly nursing service of a few visiting nurses' associations.

That many more hospital wards and health services did not have to be closed during the war for the lack of personnel is a tribute to the imagination and organizational skill demonstrated by administrators under exceedingly trying circumstances. It was tacitly assumed that once the war was over the hospitals could return to their "normal" ways, and that the voluntary hospital, at least, could get back largely to a graduate and student nurse basis. Like the producers of steel who have continuously insisted that in another six months the "emergency" demand would be over, many hospital administrators believed that presently graduate nurses would come trooping back and difficulties would end. The record since 1945 has demonstrated the error of that presumption. The bitter truth is slowly being borne in on those responsible for planning that, so great is the demand, there is no considerable body of nurses to come trooping back. Instead, they are being thinly dispersed over large geographic and occupational areas.

The task of the future therefore seems to be that of analyzing and utilizing the experience gained prior to and during the war for long-term constructive planning; of fashioning from those frequently inchoate elements a *functional* system in which, through coordination, training, and supervision, persons of many different skills may render efficient service in the area of the health services.

Objections to Extended Use of Assistant Personnel

In a 1947 pamphlet, Practical Nurses and Auxiliary Workers for the Care of the Sick, the Joint Committee on Auxiliary Nursing Service, composed of appointed representatives of six national nursing associations, committed itself unequivocally to recognition of specific functions for assistant nursing personnel. In spite of this official statement, many individual nurses speak disparagingly of the use of assistant personnel in caring for the sick. In conversations with nurses throughout the country, the writer heard two recurrent arguments which indicate sincere anxiety: in one instance, anxiety

---

* A count for January 1948, made by the National League of Nursing Education of the number of hospitals operating schools of nursing which employ practical nurses, showed that about 25 percent utilized this form of assistant nursing care.

concerning patient care; in the other, anxiety about the R.N.'s own future. Unless these fears can be allayed, the building of coordinated teams of health workers will be seriously retarded regardless of any official statements by joint committees.

Over and again directors of nursing service and nurse educators, generally employed in excellent voluntary hospitals, plead for the best in nursing service that can be provided patients. How can that best be available, they ask, other than through the exclusive use of graduate nurses? They often observe pertinently that even the giving of a bed-bath, the placing of a tray, or the drawing of a window shade may be made by the nurse into therapeutic elements in her care of an acutely sick person. They argue with absolute convincingness that the patient is, and hence should be cared for as, a complete or total person. Treatment of a localized disease or postoperative area is not enough. Treatment of the emotional component is equally important.

The reason that other persons plead for the use of a differentiated staff, particularly by the voluntary hospital that has usurped a large proportion of the supply of R.N.s, is that the best in nursing service that can possibly be provided is desired both for patients in *all* hospitals and in *homes,* and for the *public at large.* Were the personnel and funds available, such persons would like to see the finest individualized care supplied to every one, sick and well. The shortage of nurses makes it essential, in their opinion, that the existent supply be utilized more advantageously and distributed more equitably. The graduate staff nurse should be freed, or should free herself, to the maximum degree from those relatively unimportant duties still performed by her in order that she may concentrate her whole attention, within the voluntary hospital, upon the acutely ill and those in greatest need of total care. Any private duty nurse who cares for one patient not in real need of her exclusive attention, and any hospital or physician who condones or encourages that practice, render a grave injustice to society.

Nursing care in most of the public specialized hospitals and many of the public general hospitals is on an extremely elementary and unsatisfactory level. At least enough thoroughly competent graduate nurses must be found for supervision, administration, and teaching both of in-service and clinical courses, and divisions of such hospitals used for clinical instruction must be adequately staffed below the supervisory level. Unless this can be done, little hope is seen for future improvement.

Furthermore, much thought is given to those 145,000,000 persons who are not recumbent in hospital beds on a given day. Very appreciable numbers of them need the home services of visiting nurses, which are not available even in much of urban America. Still larger numbers need active help in preventing disease and maintaining health.

Finally, those persons who advocate the use of a differentiated staff are not unmindful of that realistic problem of the individual's and the institution's budget. We are still far from discovering a financial method whereby the finest in nursing could be furnished to everyone in need. At least it is assumed that neither the patient nor the institution should pay for graduate nursing, if any part of that nursing could be done as efficiently by persons with shorter preparation.

Another reason for the lack of conviction by nurses about wide preparation and utilization of assistant personnel is apparently rooted in the fear felt by many private duty nurses of the trained practical nurse. They see in her a potential competitor who is much sought after and who often earns not much less than they earn. They do not like to think about the consequences, were the current demand for private practitioners to decrease or were large numbers of practical nurses "to flood the market." Even institutional nurses are sometimes alarmed about the latter contingency. They fear, so they say, that practical nurses may "take over." They refer not only to the capture of practice but to control of nursing policies.

That some practical nurses are even now in competition with individual private duty nurses can scarcely be gainsaid. Whether enough trained practical nurses could be produced to be numerically a source of worry to the profession appears exceedingly doubtful at present. That there would be any substantial future threat from them, should they become readily available, is still more unlikely *provided graduate nurses move in the years ahead to true professional status.* The test might eventually lie in whether real differentiation of function is achieved. The writer believes that a place of such responsible leadership can and should be given to the *professional* nurse that persons with trained skill in uncomplicated general nursing would be viewed by the professional nurse and by society as essential helpers, certainly not as competitors.

Engineering an Example of Differentiated Functions

The existence side by side, within an occupation one sector of which is professional, of several kinds of persons differing rather clearly in type of preparation and function performed, but not necessarily in name, has been so little noted by most persons that first encounters with the situation are often bewildering. Hence the experience of engineering may help to illuminate thought about nursing.

In its broad scope engineering is an occupation that employs persons with varying degrees of ability and training. It has within its ranks men whose training ranges from the most advanced scientific and technological education to very little formal education. Engineering enterprises require the services of three groups of men: professional engineers, whose primary functions are planning and directing; technicians, skilled in developing details of plans and in supervision; and engineering artisans, whose manual dexterity and experience are needed to carry out plans.

Professional engineers provide the intellectual leadership in engineering. Many of them are convinced, however, that there are not yet sufficient opportunities for truly advanced preparation so that the leadership is either as profound in scientific knowledge or in its understanding of social purpose as it should be. Because attention has been primarily centered on developing a general basic education within the undergraduate engineering college that would give the essentials of professional training to matriculants, graduate curricula have not been adequately cultivated.

Engineering technicians, who are generally spoken of as engineers and thus speak of themselves, are employed on the operating level. They do not confine themselves to engineering enterprises as do many professional engineers, but enter industrial production in considerable numbers. In industry they occupy supervisory positions in operating departments; they supply such technical services as drafting, designing, testing, and inspection; they fill commercial positions relating to the sale of technical products and services. Under no circumstances should it be assumed that these technicians are men of generally lesser competence than are professional engineers. Many of them have a specialized efficiency that amazes the professional engineer as well as the laity. Their work is of unquestioned importance in the maintenance and operation of industry and in the forwarding of engineering enterprises. The scope of their work, however, is narrow, and responsibility assumed for over-all planning and administration is negligible.

Trade schools and technical high schools are designed to provide training for engineering artisans. Many learn their vocation, however, by being employed on the job or by the in-service training furnished by industry. There are a handful of excellent technical institutes that prepare a relatively small number of technicians. Unfortunately these institutes are far too few to meet the large potential demand for technicians. The course of study is generally two years in length, and students are admitted primarily on evidence of their capacity, interest, and in some instances future employability, rather than on presentation of formal scholastic credentials. All curricula are more distinctly vocational than are those of four-year engineering colleges. Yet they include a substantial amount of the underlying and related sciences and usually some work in English and economics. "Doing to learn" is an important characteristic of the instruction; a considerable portion of the student's school hours is devoted to practice in laboratories, shops, drawing, and design. The ranks of this group are supplemented by men who work up from the artisan level,

and by some graduates of engineering colleges who at least begin their practice as technicians.

The schools of engineering that confer degrees are especially designed for
the formal training of professional engineers who wish to enter the fields of
planning and management. The four-year instruction received in these schools
is supplemented, during summer vacations and after completion of the academic course, by supervised practical experience in industry. Because of an
imbalance in the proportionate numbers of engineering colleges and of technical institutes that arose from America's extreme devotion to academic degrees, relatively too many professional engineers and too few technicians have
been prepared. Since the onset of World War II, professional engineers—like
nurses—have been in urgent demand. Prior to that, however, many graduates
of engineering colleges were obliged to take positions in the technical services for which their preparation had been unnecessarily long. At all times, on
the other hand, the supply of technicians has been totally insufficient to serve
the practical direction of industry.

Building Nongraduate Personnel into Integrated
Service Teams

No one assumes that the task of creating efficient, differentiated but integrated nursing service based upon functional requisites will be easy or readily
accomplished, or that progress will everywhere be uniform. No one who
knows the diversity of conditions from hospital to hospital and from agency
to agency would advocate a single pattern or even several patterns to be
slavishly copied, regardless of suitability. What is advocated is wide experimentation, pooling and exchange of ideas, critical evaluation of accomplishment, and then further experimentation on the basis of lessons learned. What
is advocated, furthermore, as an absolute antecedent to such experimentation
is conviction, not lip-service alone, on the part of the nursing profession, the
other health professions including hospital administrators, and the laity concerned with social change, that new patterns of nursing service must be
evolved both in behalf of adequacy of supply and of quality. The elements
for these patterns, it has been seen, are largely known. They have been used
sometimes for years in differing degrees in many places. How various kinds
of personnel can be better selected and trained, and their efforts coordinated
is the problem to be solved.

Particularly instructive is an experiment now being undertaken in one
large general hospital in solving the problem of unsatisfactory ward attendants. This hospital had been much impressed by the intelligence, understanding, and interest shown by the nurse's aides who had volunteered their serv-

ices during the war. Could personnel be found and trained to replace the attendants, who would more nearly resemble these former volunteers? Public announcement was made of raised standards for application and improved wages. In response to this request for persons designated as nursing aides, the hospital discovered among the large Negro community a hitherto untapped reservoir of personnel, well above the ward attendant group in intelligence and personality. Although the hospital is in a "border" city, it decided to select aides from among these applicants. One month of carefully designed and paid in-service training was provided as preparation for work in a particular division of the hospital. The aides were then assigned to that division. They were found shortly to be doing everything formerly done by ward attendants; they were also carrying, under supervision, an appreciable number of the more routine nursing duties previously performed by graduate nurses. So successful was the initial experiment that the plan, still less than a year old, has already been extended to several other divisions.

Space permits the inclusion of only one other illustration. Consequently, we turn to an experiment in total, integrated staffing of a teaching hospital that serves primarily as a diagnostic and surgical center for difficult referred cases. In this institution differentiation according to function has been carried far toward its logical conclusion. The women's wards, for example, utilize the services of ward maids, attendants, trained practical nurses, graduate nurses for specialized aspects of bedside care, sometimes student nurses, and ward secretaries. Each ward is administered by a head nurse who has had advanced preparation for, or considerable satisfactory experience in, ward management. She will presently be aided by two assistant head nurses, one of whom will supposedly devote her time to teaching both students and the regularly employed personnel. Particularly gratifying, in the opinion of the director of nursing service, is the transformation in morale and nursing practices on the men's wards. Gone is the orderly who had been far from satisfactory. Men attendants, men trained practical nurses, and men graduate nurses have been introduced.

Throughout the hospital emphasis is placed on the role each has to play as a team in the care of patients. Deviation from that role is believed to endanger good nursing care and team relationships, and also the carefully figured budget. It has been difficult, however, to persuade some graduate nurses that they must relinquish routine duties, the practice of which has become habitual. This plan of staffing was instituted during the difficult war period. At no time has it been possible to get or retain many of the persons desired. The results have been sufficiently good, however, so that the director is now having a careful analysis made of results obtained and next steps to be taken. It is to be hoped that a detailed description of this undertaking and a report of the analysis will be published at the earliest possible moment, in order that other hospitals requiring large amounts of specialized nursing service may be able to compare practices. Obviously so elaborate a plan is not suitable for the average community hospital where most cases are less difficult of diagnosis, treatment, and nursing care.

Before turning to a few brief suggestions about procedures necessary for attracting, retaining, and increasing the efficiency of assistant personnel in general, something more specific must be said concerning the trained practical nurse around whom so many hopes and also some fears center as the potential future source of much bedside nursing. Of the nongraduate personnel, she has had the broadest and most formal preparation, although it has rarely exceeded a year in length. Perhaps because she stands closest to the R.N., fairly specific policy determinations have been reached by the nursing profession about the area of her competence.

It was the consensus of the Joint Committee on Auxiliary Nursing Service and of the six boards of directors represented by that committee that the trained practical nurse "is prepared to care for subacute, convalescent and chronic patients and to assist the registered professional nurse in the care of others. She works under the direction of a licensed physician and the supervision of the registered professional nurse. She may work in homes, hospitals, institutions, public health agencies, doctors' offices, and in commercial and industrial firms."* The Professional Advisory Committee for the present study concurred in this statement and stressed the fact that the trained practical nurse might assist in the care of acute illness as the member of a team where adequate supervision was present. Such a statement of official policy, if widely distributed and staunchly supported, should do much to give recognition to the broad scope of the work available to her, and to her place within an integrated team at least in instances of acute sickness.

Unfortunately the trained practical nurse does not yet have any appreciable legal recognition and protection, which are requisite if she is to feel much assurance or pride in her job. Before she is employed by an institution or public health agency, her training will probably be carefully questioned. In the field of home nursing that is desperately in need of many thousand more trained practical nurses, however, she must compete—except in three jurisdictions—with any person who chooses to "nurse for hire." In some 20 states legislation forbids the use of the title, licensed practical or attendant nurse, to those who have not been granted statutory permission. But anyone may put on a uniform and simply call herself a "nurse." Only in New York, Arkansas, and Hawaii have statutes been enacted which make it illegal for a person not

---

* *Practical Nurses and Auxiliary Workers for the Care of the Sick.* New York, 1947, p. 7.

a registered nurse or a licensed practical or attendant nurse to engage in nursing for pay. Under such circumstances one can imagine the chaotic conditions that prevail. The trained practical nurse who specializes in home care is likely to find that many of her colleagues in uniform are persons with no preparation and often little competence, but who succeed remarkably well in passing as "nurses" and in collecting very substantial fees.

If such lack of regulation is detrimental to the building of a large body of respected and self-respecting trained practical nurses, it is positively dangerous to society. Numerous instances are known of techniques employed and drugs administered by well-meaning but ignorant "nurses" that endangered life. For the very reason that persons of limited education are most likely to be at the mercy of such a practitioner, it is doubly important that they be provided with any possible protection which they are unable to provide for themselves. Whenever efforts are made to end this disgraceful negligence through legislative enactment, loud cries proclaim that even poor nursing is better than no nursing. There are not nearly enough veterinaries to meet current demands; yet society requires that they be licensed before they can practice. Other means than mere avoidance of needed legal action must be sought for furnishing a more adequate supply of home nursing care. *We recommend that sound legislation relating to trained practical nurses be enacted promptly in states without statutes; that such legislation elsewhere be reviewed, amended, and made mandatory as of a fixed date.**

Because this report concerns itself primarily with a very different topic, further discussion here of the practical nurse is impossible.** Attention must therefore be directed again to the total group of nongraduate personnel who perform or could be trained to perform the less complicated nursing duties. Surely the writer can offer no specific formulas for their recruitment and retention or for making them efficient in their work. Past experience nevertheless has indicated certain broad steps that must be taken if these *desiderata* are to be achieved. More careful planning and administration of policies as agreed upon should be instituted. Policies for selection, tenure, wages, duties

---

* Unfortunately space does not permit discussion in this report of legislation and administrative regulations concerning nursing practice by, and nursing education for, other types of nurses. Hence it can only be stated emphatically that statutory and administrative review, amendment, and enactment of new legislation and rulings are reported to be needed in practically every jurisdiction. Many clauses in existing acts and many interpretative rulings of state boards of nurse examiners have become so outmoded that they are a serious obstacle to much needed developments.

** Now available elsewhere, is the first detailed study of this very important subject: *The Practical Nurse* written by Dorothy Deming, R.N., consultant in public health nursing to the American Public Health Association, and published in 1947 by the Commonwealth Fund in New York.

to be performed, physical conditions of work extending to just such small but important details as adequate rest rooms, and so on, need thoughtful definition. Once determined these policies should be made generally known. If generously conceived to raise the importance and dignity of the nongraduate position, they would probably be of very appreciable help in recruiting personnel.

In-service training would unquestionably have to be fashioned into a truly effective instrumentality for initial and continuing preparation of personnel. Although it has long been used in hospitals, particularly in those which have depended largely upon attendant care of patients, there is wide consensus that its great potentialities have rarely been envisioned. Even industry, which has relied upon this form of training to no inconsiderable degree, is convinced that cultivation still falls far short of inherent possibilities.

We believe that in-service training should be at least as carefully devised and the quality of instruction as adequate as is training now given to student nurses in the typical hospital school. We believe, furthermore, that in-service training, rather than the operation of a school for the preparation of graduate nurses, should progressively come to be the essential task of the majority of hospitals. As will be argued later, other institutions can better prepare the graduate nurse than can they. At present many hospitals are sacrificing the area that they probably should cultivate assiduously to programs for student nurses which they are ill-equipped to provide.

In-service training, moreover, is needed by nearly everyone employed, graduate as well as nongraduate, on a continuing basis. Thus far its principal use has been to induct new, nongraduate personnel into their initial duties. It can provide considerable initial efficiency to be sure, but it can also be used to maintain and raise that efficiency. (Through it other evidence besides length of "satisfactory" experience is available for upgrading in salary and status, with the probable concomitant effect of producing a better satisfied as well as more efficient staff.) That in-service training, by whatever name called, is almost equally essential for graduate nurses can scarcely be denied. In a field where new scientific knowledge, new technical procedures, and new attitudes concerning the larger functions of the health services appear in rapid succession, failure to make provision for systematic examination of these developments is likely to handicap not merely the nurse but the institution or agency utilizing her services.

Perhaps most essential of all, if assistant personnel are to be recruited and retained, is the effecting of change in the emotional climate within which these persons work. So bad is that climate now in many places that the writer recalls the comment of an administrator in a representative community hospital. "We get practical nurses, they stay a few days or weeks and leave. You can scarcely blame them. They have no status. They are treated like scrub women." Unless attention can be centered squarely upon the importance of the contribution that each person brings to the health services, be that person ward maid or director of nursing service, efforts to create and stabilize a differentiated personnel will be of small avail. And unless every contributing person can be conceived of and treated as the member of a unified team, whose sole collective function is the cure of sickness and the preservation of health, we shall be little better off than at present.

We believe, therefore, that consideration should be given not only to provisions for greatly expanded and improved in-service training and for more carefully designed policies for recruitment and employment, but that primary consideration should be placed upon achieving better interpersonal relationships within the hospital.

In 1944, fifteen states had provisions for licensure of some kind of auxiliary nursing personnel; within the next few years all fifty states had licensed practical nurses, although only eight have mandatory requirements. Part of the motivation of the registered nurses who helped push these acts through the state legislatures was a desire to control the new practitioners they saw developing. On the other hand, licensure gave status and security to the new workers, as well as helped to specify their role in the developing system. As the auxiliary practitioners developed, registered nurses had to redefine their own role, and it was out of this new arrangement of roles that the concept of the "nursing team" developed. This term was first used in the report of the Committee on the Function of Nursing in *A Program for the Nursing Profession* (New York: The Macmillan Company, 1948) and was popularized by Eleanor Lambertsen, who, in 1953, published a report of research done through Teachers College, Columbia University, in which team nursing was used for patient care. *(Nursing Team Organization and Functioning)*. The organization of roles within the nursing care sub-system which she outlined came to be the model for most hospitals.

The registered nurses, however, remained ambivalent about their changing role. Though they might have extensive knowledge and great skill, they did not feel completely secure in the team situation. Lyle Saunders, the medical sociologist, emphasized this ambiguity.

18.

The Changing Role of Nurses

by Lyle Saunders

Professional training in a field such as nursing, to a considerable extent, consists in learning the behaviors that are appropriate to one or more fairly well defined roles, the ways in which those roles interlock with others in complex systems, and the skills that are necessary for at least minimum effectiveness in performance. A role, as defined by social psychologists, is not necessarily what anybody does. It is rather that complex of behavior that is expected of one who occupies a given position or office. Since roles are defined in terms of collective expectations, any considerable difference in the set of expectations one group or another has with respect to a given role may make difficult the performance of the role. If, as sometimes happens, doctors have one set of notions about what nurses should do and nurses have different ideas of what their role is, any performance is likely to produce strain, to the extent that it is not consistent with the nurses' own conception of their role or with their idea of what the physicians' expectations are.

There are, of course, many contexts within which the nursing role can be discussed. The one presented here is that of the nurse as an employee; of the nurse viewed as one type of worker among many types in a highly specialized kind of enterprise in which the raw material worked on happens to be sick human beings; of the nurse as a member of an occupational group that has been affected, as many other occupations have, by the forces of an evolving industrial society; of the nurse as a particular kind of "white collar" worker.

Now this is not a way that nurses commonly conceive of themselves. It would be difficult to say what is the most common collective image nurses have of themselves but it certainly would not be this one. They may view themselves as ministering angels, as skilled and competent technicians, as champions of the cause of comprehensive or total care, as members of a professional group battling for proper recognition and a rightful place in the therapeutic sun, or in any one of a number of other ways. They do not often, as a group, see themselves as workers, subject to many of the same forces and beset by many of the same problems that trouble workers generally in an industrial society. This is not a very glamorous view nor, I suspect, a popular one. But it is realistic, and it has many implications for the present situations in which nurses find themselves.

Reprinted, with permission, from *The American Journal of Nursing*, LIV, 1954, 1094–98.

Characteristics of Nursing As an Occupation

As an occupation, nursing has certain characteristics, some of which set it apart from other occupations, and others that identify it with other occupations.

A first characteristic is that nursing is highly diversified. People who think of themselves as nurses and are called nurses by others work at such a variety of tasks and in such a wide range of situations that it is sometimes difficult to see what they have in common. The person who receives patients in a doctor's office and sends out bills at the end of the month is a nurse; so is a woman who operates the sterilizer in a central supply department of a hospital, a head of a department in a vast insurance corporation, a dean of a college, an administrative head of a small rural hospital, an army lieutenant, a classroom teacher, a public health worker, a clinic supervisor, a ship's officer, and a dozen other categories that could be named. People are nurses whose training ranges from three or possibly fewer years spent in a hospital setting, with a minimum of formal academic instruction, to Ph.D.'s with years of both practical and theoretical training.

A second characteristic of nursing as an occupation is that it carries a somewhat ambiguous status. The training period is long and the requirements high, but the rewards are generally low and the prestige not very great. Like school teachers and social workers, nurses must have extensive knowledge, the mastery of complicated skills, and must carry a heavy responsibility. Like these other professional persons, they tend to be poorly rewarded and inadequately appreciated. It is not without significance, that even in a time of great demand for their services, the salaries of nurses remain relatively low. A part of the discrepancy between requirements and rewards may lie in lingering notions we all have about the relative capabilities of men and women. That nursing, social work, and school teaching are occupations largely followed by females may be one reason for the fact that rewards are not adequately scaled to the training required or the responsibility carried.

When we think about them in their entirety the complexity and range of the requirements of the nursing role are almost frightening. In addition to a highly developed sense of professional responsibility, the nurse is expected to have an extensive knowledge of the basic physical and biological sciences, including pharmacology; a sensitivity to the implications of an enormous variety of physical signs and symptoms; skill in the use of numerous complicated instruments and complex techniques; personal attributes of tact, sensitivity, kindness, cheerfulness, compassion, generosity, initiative, and warmth; a thorough knowledge of the total organization within which she works and of the dynamic relationships among its various parts; a skill in the handling of interpersonal and inter-group relations; and a sufficient knowledge of the principles and concepts of economics, political science, social psychology, psychiatry, sociology, cultural anthropology, and administration to enable her to handle the complicated demands of her position.

The hospital nurse must be an economist to the extent that she is concerned with the allocation and distribution of scarce commodities like time, effort, and materials. Because of her position as a link in a chain of command, because she exercises power and authority a good part of her behavior is political. Because effective performance in her role requires that she be sensitive to and able to cope with the feelings, emotions, and sentiments of those in her immediate work group, her patients, and herself, she is required to be something of a practicing psychiatrist. In the light of all the demands that are made upon her and the requirements that she must meet, the rewards of the nurse, both material and psychological, are exceedingly meager.

The ambiguous status of the role of nursing is reflected also in another set of factors. Nursing is almost the only profession, if not the only one, in which the most important decisions about what work is done and how it is to be done are made by people outside the profession. What school teachers do in their classrooms is determined by the teachers themselves, or by persons professionally trained in the field of education. Lawyers determine and control courtroom procedure and, through their positions as consultants to or members of law making bodies, have much to do with the actual writing of laws. But insofar as their function involves the care of sick people, the major decisions under which nurses work are made by doctors. Doctors, too, through their control of hospital policies and procedures exercise a considerable influence over the professional activities and working conditions of nurses.

A third aspect of nursing as an occupation is that it is relatively isolated—socially speaking. Although nurses seldom work alone anymore and most of them have jobs in highly complex organizations that bring them into frequent contact with other occupational groups, there is still a sense in which nurses are socially and psychologically isolated. A good part of their training, like that of medical students, is highly cloistered as compared with that of teachers, lawyers, engineers, social workers, and other professional groups. The nurse's contacts throughout the "practical" part of her training, and for the entire period of training for those who attend hospital schools, are largely with other nurses.

During the professional part of her training she attends classes with other nurse students, receives instruction mainly from teachers who are themselves nurses, spends considerable time in a hospital setting where she is identified as a member of a nursing group, and has relatively few opportunities for establishing meaningful professional relationships outside of nursing circles.

Even when she receives training in a hospital that is connected with a medical school, she seldom, if ever, has an opportunity to attend classes with medical students or those in training for some technical specialty related to medicine, and she almost never receives joint instruction in clinical subjects with students of medicine.

It is very striking to an outsider to see doctors and their student flocks proceeding through a ward, discussing cases, and a nurse instructor and her students working on the same ward, with no indication that either group has any awareness of the other's existence. And yet the students who are so carefully separated during their training are expected, when they enter their professional jobs, to undergo a transformation which will permit them to work together as members of a team sharing the responsibility for the care of patients. It is certainly not to be expected that physicians and nurses should receive identical training, but it would seem that somewhere in the training period an opportunity might be provided for them to become acquainted and to begin to learn how to work together effectively and harmoniously.

The occupational isolation of nurses is not confined to the training period. As graduate nurses, they tend to form a somewhat closed group from which outsiders are excluded. To some extent this is a natural phenomenon that is to be expected. Nurses are drawn together by common interests, common identifications, common problems. But the observable degree of isolation seems greater than could be accounted for by this alone.

It may be that the nurses have too much status, too much professional identification to be comfortable with those below them in the job hierarchy and not enough to permit easy association with the physicians who outrank them. Whatever the reasons, nurses tend, insofar as it is possible in the type of situation in which they work to associate considerably more with each other than with members of any other occupational group. In a hospital which I have had some opportunity to observe, nurses eat together, take their coffee breaks together, meet formally in a great variety of groupings to which even the subprofessional people who work closely with them and under their supervision are not invited, and plan their programs and activities almost as if they were the only group working in the institution. This practice makes for poor working relationships and may at times adversely affect the welfare of the patients, and to the extent that it exists it is something that nurses perhaps should take steps to correct.

A fourth characteristic of nursing as an occupation is that it is conservative. Nurses are not, on their jobs, brash innovators or daring experimenters. And this is perhaps both understandable and desirable in the light of the fact that the comfort, well-being and, at times, even the very lives of people may be at stake. Conservatism, dependability, stability, caution are characteristics that nurses are encouraged to develop during their period of professional socialization; attributes such as imagination, resourcefulness, progressiveness, and a liking for change are discouraged.

The conservatism that is "trained into" nurses is shown in their reluctance to take on new functions and abandon old ones; in their acceptance of rigid hospital traditions which deny them any but the smallest measure of initiative; in the suspicion with which they look upon such newcomers as aides and practical nurses; and in their tendency to cling to old routines long after they no longer serve a useful purpose.

A fifth, and highly important, characteristic of nursing is that it is organized. By far the largest proportion of today's nurses work in hospitals or similar institutions where they function as parts of complex organizations. An organization is essentially a social system—a set of positions for which functions and relationships are specified and prescribed. Individuals in organizations are assumed to be interchangeable and expendable. The important thing is the position; it must be activated by somebody, but who that somebody is does not matter much if he or she possesses the necessary knowledge and skill to fill the position. In its dynamic aspects, organization involves the relating of many persons, materials, and techniques in particular ways for the purpose of achieving certain ends.

Large scale organizations, such as those in which many nurses work, frequently possess the characteristics of bureaucracies, particular kinds of organizations in which the positions are arranged rationally in a job hierarchy in terms of differences in functions, status, authority, responsibility, and reward. Bureaucratic organization usually involves a minute division of labor, the delegation of authority and responsibility, indirect lines of communication, and a fairly high degree of authoritarianism in decision making. A bureaucratic organization is a very fine way of getting things done. It is efficient; it permits the effective use of highly specialized skills; it is economical. But it has some disadvantages too. By its uneven distribution of rewards and authority it fosters dissatisfactions; it has no place for the expression of individuality; it requires impersonal, segmental relationships; it subordinates people to a system; it acts as a mold into which occupational groups must be made to fit.

Fortunately or unfortunately, depending on the point of view, the bureaucratic type of organization suffers from the fact that it has to operate with people. If any given organization were well thought out and if all the positions could be filled by precisely trained incumbents, with no other roles and no nonoccupational interests, the system conceivably might work very well. But incumbents are not perfectly trained. Some are overtrained for the positions they hold; some are undertrained. Some lack capacity for the jobs they have; others are temperamentally unsuited for the tasks they are asked to perform. Many are dissatisfied with the rewards of their position and have their eyes on better ones.

Also, nearly everybody has a series of other roles which interfere with his occupational one. Everybody is husband or wife, son or daughter, golfer, bowler, church member, crusader, student, zealot, or whatnot and, as such, has roles which interfere with the perfect performance of his job. The attitudes, feelings, sentiments, beliefs, of these other roles are carried over into the work situation where they frequently interfere with the smooth functioning of the bureaucratic organization. The imperfect training for roles and the seeking of individual or group ends, other than those provided for in the formal organization, result in the development of a series of informal relationships whose functioning crosscuts, facilitates, hampers, and sometimes even cancels the efforts of the formal organization. Cliques form; interest groups develop; personalities clash; individuals behave from distorted ideas of their proper role and function; animosities and hostilities develop; channels for tension release are developed.

And into all of this nurses fit. Regardless of their training, regardless of their collective image of themselves, they, like everybody else, are drawn into the machinery of the bureaucratic structure and are tumbled about by it. And to a much larger extent than many of them realize, the professional problems they face, the worries they have, the frustrations they feel, the dissatisfactions that bother them are traceable to the fact of their participation in an organized occupational system.

A final point to be made about nursing as an occupation is that it is changing. And the rate and direction of change are possibly largely outside the control of nurses themselves. The past fifty years have been years of moving away from a concentration on sick people to a concentration on the mechanical and technical aspects of therapy and care. They have witnessed the change of the nurse from a self-employed entrepreneur to a salaried employee; from a person who worked largely alone and self directed to one who shares in a minute and highly specialized division of labor; from one whose relationships with those she worked among were close, intimate, and personal to one whose working relationships with both patients and colleagues are subjected to strong pressures toward becoming both impersonal and segmental; from one whose skills and functions were generalized, to one whose skills and functions are very highly specialized.

Unlike her colleague of thirty years ago, today's nurse sells her skills to an institution in return for a fixed salary. Hours of work are limited to 40 or 45 a week and almost no one regularly works more than an 8-hour shift. The nurse works with other nurses rather than alone, and in situations in which there is a fairly rigid division of labor. Instruments and appliances are more numerous and vastly more complex than they were thirty years ago, and they tend to be owned by the institution. The place of work and the conditions of work are controlled by the organization. Working relations are relatively impersonal.

The patient, largely stripped of the symbols and signs of his normal roles, is seen in an artificial setting far from his usual habitat. His care is the joint responsibility of a staff of nurses and auxiliaries. Each nurse must divide her time and attention among a large number of patients. The quality, rate, and efficiency of the nurse's work are subject to constant scrutiny. Authority and responsibility are not always clear, since a number of occupational groups are involved in the therapeutic situation and it is not always easy to know where one's area of responsibility begins and another's ends. Increasingly nurses are being drawn into a variety of tasks, many of which have little or no direct or immediate connection with the care of patients. As someone has said, "The present function of the graduate nurse is not to nurse the patient, but to see that he is nursed."

As nurses have moved away from the bedside and have increasingly taken over the function of supervising rather than giving direct nursing care, it has been necessary to create a number of new categories of subprofessional and nonprofessional workers and to recruit and train people to fill these positions. The responsibility for much of the on-the-job training and supervision of these newcomers has fallen to the professional nurses, bringing new problems, the need for new skills, and the necessity of establishing new types of relationships in the work situation.

No nurse or group of nurses can do very much alone anymore. Their professional activities make up part of a complex institutional situation in which what anyone and everyone does must be delicately adjusted to the expectations and actions of everyone else. Although the patient still remains ostensibly the center of the whole activity, a good deal of the attention of nurses must be diverted from the patient and toward other aspects of the situation. The social machinery of which nursing is a part requires attention and effort if it is to function smoothly, so that much of what nurses do is concerned more with the institutional aspects of their work routines than with giving direct attention to patients.

There is evidence that nurses, both individually and collectively, are somewhat ambivalent in their feelings about the widening gap between themselves and patients and the changing roles they are expected to assume. On the one hand they have invented or reaffirmed ideologies about their responsibility for giving "total patient care," "comprehensive nursing care," and "tender loving care" and the importance of being concerned with the "total patient," which seek to recapture and revitalize the image of the nurse as a technically competent, affect-dispensing mother substitute.

On the other hand, schools of nursing have realistically attempted to introduce into their training programs content and experiences that will enable their graduates to handle comfortably and capably the whole range of demands that their jobs will make upon them. The recent emphases in nursing curriculums on the social sciences, on understanding the dynamics of social situations, on the development and exercise of leadership skills, on the handling of interpersonal and intergroup relations, and on the principles and techniques of administration reflect not only aspirations for what nurses and nursing may become, but also an adjustment to the reality of what the nursing role now is.

It is unlikely that present trends in the direction of change in nursing are likely soon to be reversed. The high level of technical competence required of nurses, the imperatives of the hospital work situation, the relative scarcity of adequately trained people, the broad trends in medicine itself make very improbable any return to the nursing conditions of thirty years ago. The gap between nurses and patients is likely to continue to widen; more and more it is going to be the responsibility of professional nurses to see that the patient is nursed rather than to do the nursing; and the already large managerial aspect of the nursing role is almost certain to increase at the expense of more traditional elements of that role.

One result of the rapid changes that have taken place in nursing is a fairly widespread uncertainty about what properly is the nurse's role, an uncertainty that is reflected in the increasing number of studies of nursing functions and staffing patterns that are being undertaken with the encouragement and support of the American Nurses' Association.

This uncertainty is shown, too, in the deep and sometimes bitter disagreement that still exists between proponents of hospital and university training for nurses; in the tensions that can be observed between nurses and other occupational groups in some institutional settings; and in the deliberations of nurse educators about what needs to be included in the nursing curriculum. These are all evidence that no one is very certain any more what a nurse is or what a nurse properly should do.

Although it may be uncomfortable to those in nursing and nurse education, there is nothing particularly unhealthy from a sociological point of view in the present unsettled status of nursing. A series of professional role modifications are occurring. Functions are being transferred from one group to another. Privileges and responsibilities are being reshuffled and reallocated. Status lines are being shifted. All of this, although it is possibly unpleasant for those who experience it, is quite natural and perhaps inevitable in a period of rapid technological change.

New Aspects of the Nursing Role

What seems to be emerging rather clearly from the changes that have occurred and are continuing is the increasing managerial or administrative aspect of that role. For better or worse, and whether they like it or not, nurses —particularly graduates of university schools and those with special or advanced training—are being drawn into positions that, wholly or in large part, require the performance of an administrative function. Nurses have become and increasingly are becoming managers—persons whose job requires that they oversee and coordinate the work of other people. This is probably true of staff nurses, many of whom now direct and assume responsibility for the work of nonprofessional assistants. It is certainly true in hospitals for head nurses and those of higher status, as well as for many industrial nurses, nursing service executives, public health nurses, and others outside the hospital setting.

It is probably significant that in the whole area of nursing interest and activity, the jobs with the smallest rewards and the lowest status are those which center most closely in the actual care of patients, whereas those with the highest status, the largest rewards, the most desirable privileges are those farthest removed from direct contact with patients. The highest, most nearly sacred value in the professional ideology of nursing is the welfare of the individual patient. This is a value which is emphasized and affirmed over and over again throughout the student nurses' training period, in the articles that nurses write for each other, and in the discussions that nurses have with each other about their profession. It is accepted without question that the highest function of a nurse is to give compassionate, tender, personal, and technically competent care to sick people.

And yet it is quite obvious that, however high this ideal may stand in the ideological value hierarchy, it is given considerably less weight in the reality situation in which nurses work. There may be and undoubtedly is for many nurses a considerable psychological satisfaction in doing a good job of bedside nursing, but the more tangible—and presumably more highly valued rewards of the nursing profession: higher salaries, recognition, prestige, authority, esteem, deference—all these go mainly to the nurses whose functions are largely or entirely administrative or managerial.

If nurses are going to be managers, and it is quite obvious that they are, there are perhaps two or three things that they might profitably do. One is to recognize the fact and take steps to bring their feelings and attitudes into line with this new aspect of their role. They could come to some understanding with themselves and each other about what is their proper area of responsibility and performance. They could recognize that area for what it is, a highly important and useful segment of the total effort of both preventive and clinical medicine, and stop being envious of and encroaching on the doctor's function on one side and reluctant to release functions to less skilled people on the other.

They could recognize that the supervision of care of the patient is a job that is fully as important and immeasurably more demanding than the actual giving of that care, and they could develop some new images of themselves that are more realistic than the ones some of them have had in the past. They could redefine their professional function to the point where they could come to see themselves as managers and be proud of that fact. On the immediately practical side they could, as they have already started to do, learn and use more effectively and assuredly than they do now the techniques of administration for the more certain attainment of their job ends. They could make better use of the techniques of politics for the pursuit of their professional goals.

They could give students a better and more realistic preparation for the jobs they are going to hold. They could do more than they now are doing to promote and aid the recruitment and training of sub-professional assistants. Finally, as managers and people of status in the organizations in which they function, they could work more vigorously for the incorporation into the clinical routines of that body of constructive practices and attitudes which they call comprehensive care and which, if adopted, might go far toward restoring dignity, individuality, and a sense of worth in many patients and returning the true nursing function to its proper place.

The function of nurses in the past has been highly important. Their emerging role can be even more significant if, by combining old values with new techniques, they can bring its full potentialities to realization. But those potentialities can be developed only if nurses can free themselves from some of their ties with the past and can move toward their collective future with assurance, with confidence in both their aspirations and their abilities, and—equally important for success—with flexibility in the acceptance and use of new means for attaining their personal and professional goals.

As team nursing developed, much of the sustaining bedside care was delegated to the practical nurse and the nurse's aide. The registered nurse in turn took over the more complex therapeutic functions and the supervision and coordination of other practitioners. While registered nurses still give direct beside care, it is usually to the very ill patient whose needs demand a high level of technical nursing skill. The head nurse in the hospital ward is almost completely involved in supervising and coordinating the work on the unit; she also takes care of all sorts of negotiations and relationships with other hospital sub-systems. Her task, and to some extent the task of the other nurses who help coordinate care, is made more difficult by the fact that nursing comes under two distinct chains of command at the same time: that of the physician and that of the nursing administrative hierarchy. These problems are discussed in papers 19 and 20.

19.

Nursing Dilemmas in the Organization of Patient Care

by Hans O. Mauksch

Careful observation and study of the nurse's work on the patients' care unit, and my experiences as sociologist in the nursing department of a large urban hospital have led me to some interesting hypotheses.

Certain factors appear to make the position of the nurse on the patient care unit one of distinct stress and dilemmas. A look at the hospital and at the work organization from her vantage point is the focus of this discussion.

Work and Traffic

Formal, as well as the informal, relationships, pressures, and expectations affect the nurse who works at the patient's bedside. First of all, there appear to be three major categories of people on the unit.

The patients are on the unit more or less permanently; they do not, at least officially, take part in the work processes. On the contrary, they are the

Reprinted, with permission, from *Nursing Outlook, V,* 1957, 31–33.

object and objective of the hospital's human structure. In considering the nurse's position, however, we must recognize that patients represent a real source of pressure on her by voicing demands, expectations, and attitudes, and by being able to invoke the power of the medical or administrative hierarchy in case they are displeased.

The nursing service group includes professional nurses, practical nurses, student nurses, and such auxiliary personnel as clerks, nursing aides, and maids. This group is distinguished by the fact that its members are *assigned* to the patients' care unit, and that they generally stay in that work area for a consecutive workday. It is distinguished further from most other groups in the hospital in that its members have continuity of contact with the patients, with the ensuing over-all responsibility.

A large segment of the *other hospital personnel* who descend on the patient care unit to perform specific functions comprise the third group. (This does not include visitors, a group by themselves, who often help to make the patients' care unit look like a busy railroad terminal.) Among these hospital personnel who come and go on the unit are several distinct categories.

Most important are the *physicians* who appear in order to direct and determine the patients' medical care. They, and representatives of the nursing hierarchy, account for the two main groups who have the formal power of directing and influencing the work performed by the nursing force on the unit.

In addition, various members of the *paramedical services* appear on the unit to perform tasks at the patient's bedside. The number and specialization of these technicians has mushroomed during the last few years, adding to the complexity of coordinating patient care.

And last, a number of other hospital functionaries come to the patients' unit to service the physical plant or to furnish supplies and equipment.

Organization and Responsibility

In considering the traffic and organization revolving around the patients' unit, we shall consider only two basic factors and their implications. The first of these arises from the fact that the nurse is assigned to the patients' care unit and remains there while all other workers come and go. This implies that she is charged with responsibility for the totality and continuity of the patients' care.

All other persons, with the exception of the physician, are responsible only for the specific task they perform at the moment. The nurse is responsible, is accountable, is blamed, and is pressured when the complex mosaic of responsibilities relating to the care of an individual patient does not fit together properly.

The dietitian is responsible for the patient's food and its preparation. The nurse, however, is responsible for his eating it, and is the one who relays—and, therefore receives—any blame if the feeding process should go awry. This unique responsibility-blame pattern applies to the nurse for the functioning of every technician and therapist.

Although the physician assumes total responsibility for the welfare of his particular patients—much of which he delegates to the nurse—the nurse, herself, is the only one who has responsibility for the entire hospital unit. It is *her* unit. Before we consider the organization implications of this arrangement there is a psychological aspect to consider.

Human beings have a need to identify with their work product; this identification—a certain possessive relationship to the work situation—was recognized even in the days of the medieval guilds, but we tend to forget it today. Yet, the nurse who thinks of the unit as "hers" must feel frustrated by the frequent "interferences and visitations" which beset her daily routine. These visits do not merely interrupt the work flow. Few, if any, of the functionaries who appear on the unit give the nurse the recognition of being the "custodian" of this unit, and the coordinator of all its activities.

To this we can add another dilemma. The physician is responsible for the treatment of *his* patient. He prescribes and directs what the nurse is to do, and a unit with 30 or 40 patients may have as many as 10 to 15 physicians who write orders. It is up to the nurse to coordinate and to mediate among these many work pressures, since she cannot always accommodate all of them.

In order to evaluate this point properly, we must add the second of our basic factors which affect the work structure of the hospital. Every social institution exists in order to perform certain functions. As the school exists to teach, the hospital exists to care for the sick.

Once an institution is established, it must be concerned not only with the fulfillment of its function but also with the management of self-maintenance and administration. The teacher must keep order in the class before he can transmit knowledge. The mother must sew, wash dishes, and make beds, as well as provide love for her children.

Administration and Coordination

In practically all institutions, the same functionary has a responsibility to perform the basic as well as the managerial function. Not so in the hospital; here the basic function, which may be called the clinical function, lies in the hands of the physician. It is his prerogative—within limits of law and ethics—to prescribe and direct the care of the patient. The administration of the hospital, the managerial function, is in the hands of an administrator and his staff.

If we look to the patients' care unit, the head nurse and her staff are responsible for the performance of most clinical tasks, and they are also, as managers of the unit, the custodians and administrators of the work. Therefore, they receive their direction from two different, and often inadequately coordinated, channels.

Administrative policy is channeled to the head nurse via the hierarchy of the nursing department: the management of personnel, and the care of facilities, equipment, and supplies is her responsibility toward her superiors in nursing. Medical care of the patient is relayed via the echelons of the medical group: attending physicians, residents, and interns. Thus, the head nurse has two sets of bosses, and sometimes they do not coordinate.

He who has two bosses has none, and the head nurse has more than two. While the nursing department gives the head nurse one boss—the supervisor —the medical staff imposes its orders through many individual physicians, each of whom varies slightly in the type and manner of demands he imposes on her. She must accommodate all of them, and, in addition to the many attending physicians, in a teaching hospital there may be several members of the house staff who write orders for one patient.

Without the formal power to do so, but informally expected to, the nurse assumes responsibility to mediate, coordinate, and safeguard the continuity, compatibility, and even propriety of the medical care prescribed. In many interviews and observations we have discovered incidences in which the attending physician expected the nurse to discover the errors made by a member of the house staff.

Strains and Stresses

We have seen, first, how the nurse is exposed to the complexities and pressures on her work area, and, second, how she is placed in the position of having to coordinate and mediate the flow of diverse directives and orders. We might ask whether this situation is more serious today than it was and, if so, why this might be. It appears that the modern development of hospital practice has made the job of the nurse—especially the head nurse—more difficult than it was in the past.

On the basis of these findings, we think we can safely say that in the entire range of human occupational pursuits there is hardly a work situation to be found to compare in complexity and built-in frustrations with that in which the head nurse must function. Few persons have so many responsibilities with so little power.

We have no desire to place blame, however. Rather, we must analyze the factors which create this situation. The physician who puts pressure on the nurse to give the most and the best care to *his* patients is doing his job and is not aware that he is competing with others for her time. Neither he nor the administrator is always aware of the conflicts which they create for the nurse who has to satisfy both.

The nurse "belongs" to the nursing department; yet, her superiors are not always around. The physician's informal power is greater by virtue of his prestige, his physical presence, and his presence in large numbers. He may not always be aware of the fact that the patient might be using him to put pressure on the nursing force, and he may act and speak before he sees the total picture.

There is little communication between the occupational groups who work side by side in the hospital. They have learned little about each other, and, in particular, they understand little about the workers in the "lower" categories. Such communication, such understanding, is essential if the hospital is to be an efficient work community, and if the nurse is to be relieved from serving as the catchall of all troubles.

To sum it up, hospital administrators and physicians must recognize several changed factors:

1. The hospital is a more complex work community than it was formerly.

2. The separation of clinical responsibility from administrative responsibility—between medical practitioner and professional administrator—has placed the nurse in the position of representing, to patients and other staff members, administration and medicine at the same time.

3. The disappearance of the older, motherly head nurse alters certain modes for coping with the tensions of the head nurse's position. Frequently, the older nurse—who knew the attending physicians when they were residents, and who had the status accorded a mother figure—has given way to a younger, but better prepared, woman. They may handle the formal aspects of the job superbly, but, as young, frequently attractive women, they do not present symbols of authority to men in our society.

In order to remedy some of the inadequacies presented briefly here, the head nurse must be prepared to be the coordinator and administrator, which, in fact, she is. She must be prepared to accept and to use the power which her position demands, and she must be accorded this power by the institution, both formally and informally.

The medical profession must be introduced to the changing concept and scope of the head nurse's job and must learn to accept her in the hospital as a central functionary with areas of independent responsibilities, prerogatives, and privileges.

20.

Is Comprehensive Nursing Care a Realistic Goal?

by Mary E. Brackett and Joan R. Fogt

What is comprehensive nursing care? Are such familiar phrases as "nursing the whole patient," "total nursing care," and "adapting care to the needs of the individual patient," inclusive enough? Do nursing service administrators who consider comprehensive nursing a desirable goal—and most of them undoubtedly do—actually strive to attain it? Are schools of nursing preparing students to give it?

At Hartford Hospital, we explored what we meant by comprehensive nursing care, and set up the following statements to help guide us in giving such care:

1. Professional nurses are responsible for nursing care of patients.

2. The nursing provided is in compliance with the medical orders and medical care plans, and coordinates functions and activities of the other health disciplines as they contribute to the achievement of total medical care.

3. The patient is recognized as an individual, and his care is adapted to his individual needs and demands.

4. The patient receives supportive nursing care—mental, physical, spiritual, and emotional—providing for rest, security, good hygiene, and comfort.

5. The patient is encouraged and assisted by nursing toward his goal of rehabilitation as he achieves the degree of independence consistent with his medical condition.

6. The patient and his family are informed of the nursing needs he will have after discharge from the hospital, and either are given instruction necessary to provide safe and effective care or are assisted in securing continuing nursing through the proper health agency.

As an illustration of how we strive toward the goal implied in these statements, we'll present Mr. Peters, a patient with coronary heart disease, resentful at being an invalid. He rebels against having everything done for him, is frightened but will not admit it, fights the oxygen, and worries about his family. The doctor leaves many orders, is thoughtful in giving the nurses information about Mr. Peters and his family, and relies on the nurses to coordinate the many facets of his plan of care.

What will the nurse, oriented to our concept of comprehensive nursing care, do for Mr. Peters? She will give him hygienic care, see that he gets his medications and treatments and, while doing this, will try to gain his confidence. She will listen to him in order that she may learn what he is like,

Reprinted, with permission, from *Nursing Outlook*, IX, 1961, 402–404.

what he fears, what he expects, what worries him. She will try to analyze what she observes, and plan accordingly. For instance, if she sees that Mr. Peters resists being waited upon hand and foot, she will not force attention upon him. She will know that it is better for him to have no bath today than to have one which upsets him emotionally. In other words, she will try to modify her nursing care to meet his needs rather than to impose hospital routines upon him.

She will make an effort to talk with and to know Mrs. Peters, and share with her information she should have; she will seek her help in dealing with Mr. Peters' individual characteristics. She will communicate with other nurses and nursing personnel caring for Mr. Peters so that the nursing he receives will be consistent and continuous. She will work skillfully as she cares for him in the oxygen tent, planning so that the concentration of oxygen will be kept constant and uninterrupted by unnecessary tent openings. She will plan with the laboratory and x-ray departments so that their work with Mr. Peters will result in minimum fatigue to him.

If he complains about his low sodium diet, she will be sympathetic, not critical. She will find out what food he likes and will ask the dietitian to prepare a diet more appealing to him. She will ask members of other disciplines, such as the social worker and the chaplain, for help if she feels there is need for them. She will, with guidance from the doctor, help Mr. and Mrs. Peters prepare for his return home and may be instrumental in getting him referred to a visiting nurse service.

This brief resumé emphasizes the fact that comprehensive nursing is not like an assembly line in a factory. It cannot be performed by robots who can be taught to do the same thing in the same way day after day. Higher than average intelligence is required to do essential, thoughtful planning; keen initiative is needed to make reasonable adjustments of the plan; and discriminating judgments are necessary to select from all observations and reactions those which are of most importance to the patient's welfare.

Comprehensive nursing is not easily attained. Many barriers make its accomplishment difficult. First, there is the hospital situation with its problem of large numbers of patients and shortage of staff. Set routines for meals, maid service, laboratory tests, doctors' rounds; and close schedules in x-ray, operating room, and physical medicine are frequently encountered. How can the nurse sit and listen to the patient who needs to talk, when a doctor wants someone (the nurse) to assist him with a patient who has just gone into cardiac arrest, or when another patient requires alternating tourniquets, and still another must have frequent blood pressure readings?

In other words, how can the nurse get to know as individual human beings all of the patients who are assigned to her? How can the nurse fit the hospital meal-time to the patient's needs when breakfast is served at 7:30 A.M. sharp, and her patient did not get to sleep until 4:30 A.M.? How can she provide for his rest when his room must be cleaned according to a strict schedule? How can she coordinate the laboratory work with x-ray examinations so that her patient's breakfast will not be withheld twice when once would suffice?

A second factor making comprehensive nursing care difficult is that the nurse may lack the essential skills for providing comprehensive nursing to one or more patients. Unfortunately, some nurses are graduates of schools which make no attempt to teach comprehensive nursing. To them, nursing consists of getting baths given, medications administered, and treatments done. Others graduate from schools where comprehensive nursing is provided by nurses alone. Throughout their programs, these nurses' assignments have been limited to the number of patients for whom it would be possible to give really comprehensive nursing care, sometimes giving care to only one patient. When they accept employment in a busy hospital and are assigned as team leaders to care for a large number of patients with the assistance of licensed practical nurses and nursing aides, their frustrations are almost unbearable. The pressures of the work situation have caused still other nurses, who learned comprehensive nursing as students, to lower their standards.

On one hand, therefore, we find registered nurses with no practical knowledge of comprehensive care but who are well adjusted to routine assembly line nursing, and on the other hand, registered nurses well equipped with knowledge and skill essential to giving comprehensive nursing to one patient, but totally unprepared to deal with many.

We find ourselves, therefore, in the position of accepting comprehensive nursing care as a desirable and worth-while goal, but confronted by a reality that makes achievement of the goal seem almost hopeless. After 12 years of struggle, frustration, and some solid accomplishment in our hospital, we continue to feel that team nursing is one useful approach to making the goal realistic as well as desirable.

Comprehensive nursing care, for most patients, requires the skills of the professional nurse. We all know, however, that many of the patient's needs can be met by less skilled persons. This knowledge and the permanent shortage of professional nurses, establishes the inevitability of using a variety of workers in nursing. In team nursing, these persons work in a close relationship with a professional nurse team leader. She retains the responsibility for the care of a larger group of patients than she could care for alone. Thus, a maximum number of patients benefit from her ability to make their care comprehensive.

Because a team leader is more accessible to both the patient and the nursing aide than the head nurse is, she is in an advantageous position to make observations, direct, evaluate, and participate in the care needed. The team conference, essential to successful team nursing, makes a unique contribution toward achieving comprehensive nursing care. Frequently, as a result of this device—which provides an opportunity for communication and problem solving—we have seen an increase in understanding and a broadened scope of care.

One natural outcome of the team conference has been written nursing care plans, another step toward our goal. Even the simplest and briefest plan has value. A written record of nursing needs, with plans and approaches for meeting these needs, helps the team keep its thinking and attention focused in the direction of comprehensive nursing care. The written plan contributes to continuity of care, and encourages the evaluation of the care given. This leads to satisfaction when the approach has been successful, and to a new plan when unsuccessful.

The difficulties involved in translating this fine theory into accomplished fact are considerable. Some head nurses find it very hard to relinquish any of their responsibilities. Some anticipate a diminution of their power and resent team nursing for this reason. Some find it difficult to stand by while the team leader performs tasks less effectively than they themselves would. An experienced head nurse can make out the day's work assignment with skill and dispatch. The young team leader has less awareness of all the factors involved and less judgment to apply to those she does recognize. Unless the head nurse accepts the philosophy and principles of team nursing, this "early morning frustration" may cause considerable resentment.

But, it is to the team leader that team nursing presents the biggest threat and the greatest challenge—as well as an opportunity for much satisfaction. The young nurse does not have sufficient knowledge of nursing or leadership skill to feel secure in this role. Regardless of what her basic preparation has been, she needs help, as a beginning practitioner, if she is to become an effective team leader. Lack of understanding of the great amount of teaching, support, and supervision she needs probably has caused team nursing to fail in many places.

We have tried many programs and approaches, and it is our firm conviction that, in spite of the difficulties, it is possible to help team leaders function effectively and take pride and pleasure in this kind of responsibility. In our experience, team members (student nurses, nursing aides, and licensed practical nurses) welcome team nursing without reservation. They appreciate both the psychological and physical accessibility of the team leader. Their feeling of worth and belonging is enhanced by participation in the team conference. In a recent poll, almost all reported that they find team conferences and nursing care plans helpful. Their chief complaint was the inadequate number of conferences and nursing care plans.

Even though team nursing can move us one giant step toward our goal of comprehensive nursing care, the fact remains that for most of us there just is not enough time to do what we know needs to be done. Because this is true, we must think in terms of priorities. If only we could teach our team leaders, and through them the team members, to concentrate on and emphasize, and be constantly aware of the things that are most important to the patient's welfare. We have struggled for years to free ourselves from a ritualistic, authoritarian, task-oriented approach, but we still have a long way to go. Certainly, the values and comfort to the patient of clean skin, tidy hair, and a wrinkle-free bed are not to be minimized, and hygienic care is still, in general, one of the highest priority items in the patient's nursing care. But, we rarely see a patient who is unclean today—and we often see patients who are fearful, lonely, untaught, uncooperative.

The nurse may not have time to sit at the bedside of the apprehensive patient for a half hour and explore his fears. If the team leader is performing effectively, however, she will know that a patient needs help and will see that he gets it. She will make herself available to him while she is performing some part of his physical care, or she will assign his care to the person best prepared to provide the support needed. She will see this as a high priority need and provide for it in some manner.

Circumstances may make it impossible for the head nurse to arrange a multidiscipline conference so that a really good plan may be made for the care of a patient who has diabetes with complications and a problem social situation. If the nurse has the ability and interest to make an accurate assessment of the patient's needs, however, she can find some way to bring the social worker and the dietitian into the picture, and to coordinate their efforts.

All nursing personnel need help in learning how to determine priorities. They need guidance and support in the nursing unit where they are giving care. Frequently, the only persons with sufficient experience to give this help are the head nurse and the supervisor. If administrative duties make it impossible for them to give sufficient guidance to team leaders perhaps a clinical specialist should be available to perform this function. Effective use of an administrative assistant to the head nurse might free the head nurse to give the needed guidance to the team.

The dilemma we face in accepting comprehensive nursing care as a goal needs to be understood by all. Every student must be thoroughly prepared to give comprehensive nursing care; she also needs to begin to learn how to establish priorities; she needs experiences which will help her find satisfaction in accepting comprehensive nursing care as it relates to a group of patients. As a young practitioner, the nurse must be helped constantly to maintain her goal of comprehensive nursing care, and to increase her skill in establishing priorities of care.

It is very important, too, for head nurses and supervisors to be aware of the fact that staff nurses are bound to suffer some frustration because of the disparity between the ideal which they have been taught and the reality of the nursing situation they confront almost daily. Many succumb to the frustration by abandoning the goal or by leaving the field. Perhaps a greater recognition of their frustration would help. They need opportunity to express their feelings. Nursing service supervisors and administrators should be constantly alert for opportunities to express understanding and support for the staff nurses who so often carry a large workload. Many nurses feel that nursing and hospital administrators are unaware of the problems they are facing. They think that the administrators are so remote from the patient's bedside that they naturally minimize the difficulties encountered there.

Good human relations will not make a nurse happy about an unreasonable workload. But if she can see that administration knows when the load is unreasonable, actively works for improvement, and seeks her participation and suggestions to help solve the problems, she will, at least, find the situation more tolerable.

Hospital nursing service administrators look to nurse educators to prepare nurses for today's world. Statistics show that more graduate nurses are employed in hospital nursing services than in any other area. It seems reasonable, therefore, to expect schools to prepare students for the kind of care hospital nursing services desire to give—nursing patterned to meet the needs of individual patients yet possible within the limitations of staff and funds.

Perhaps an analogy could be made with teaching school. Undoubtedly, educators in programs preparing teachers for public schools would like to feel that the young graduate will have her first teaching experience in a class limited to the optimum number of students. Yet, the realities of the population increase dictate that the new teacher's first class will exceed what is, theoretically, an optimum number. Should her educational program, then, prepare her to deal only with the optimum number of pupils, leaving the employing agency to carry the responsibility, through inservice education, for helping her to meet the actual teaching situation? Likewise, should the school of nursing prepare the nurse only to care for the number of patients to whom she alone can give individualized care, leaving the responsibility to the employing agency, through inservice education, to teach her to lead a team of auxiliary workers and determine priorities in individualizing care for a large group of patients? Should the nursing school teach only the responsibility of giving care to patients for eight hours of the day, and leave it to nursing service, through inservice programs, to prepare the young graduate to recognize the needs and care for the patients during the other two-thirds of their hospital day?

Our hope is that schools of nursing will assume responsibility for preparing nurses to be team leaders capable of giving nursing care to patients at any hour of the day, and capable of comprehending and planning for the fulfillment of the needs of a fairly large number of patients with a comparatively small staff.

Such preparation does not lessen the need for nursing services to develop inservice education programs that start on employment, to determine the needs of new staff members, and to provide for fulfillment of these needs. Even though the nursing student has begun to learn to be a team leader, once she has graduated, she must learn the responsibilities of team leadership at X hospital. Even though she understands comprehensive nursing, she must learn to what degree it is possible and how it is achieved at this hospital. Even though she has an idea of the responsibilities of the charge, evening, and night nurses, she must learn the responsibilities of these tours of duty at X hospital.

We hope, also, that programs preparing clinical nursing specialists will thrive, and that employment of these persons in a staff relationship, relieved of administrative duties, will be accepted by nursing services.

There is little doubt that nursing service administrators and hospital administrators need to analyze activities of nursing personnel and other hospital departments providing direct care to patients, to determine if the goal of comprehensive care is being achieved. If it is not, further studies should be done to see what reallocation of responsibilities and change of routine will make the desired goal attainable.

We see the responsibility for making comprehensive nursing a realistic goal as resting on the collective shoulders of hospital administrators, nursing service administrators, and nursing educators. Recognition of joint responsibility is a first step toward finding the way.

What then is the role of the nurse in the changing nursing situation? Nurses themselves are not agreed on what their new role should be. From the rather extensive literature the following four different answers have been selected.

21.
What Is Good Nursing Care?

by Frances Reiter Kreuter

What is good nursing care? As I asked myself this question, I went to the statement that "nursing is one of the services for the care of the sick, the prevention of illness and the promotion of health, which is carried out under medical authority."* I agree with this, but I think I would qualify the last clause, "a portion of which is carried out under medical authority."

Nursing care is a component of nursing practice. Other components of nursing practice are: *coordinating* nursing care with the care of the medical and allied professional practitioners; *planning* for continuity of care in home, school, industry, clinic, as outpatient or inpatient in hospitals, with other nurse practitioners; *evaluating* total patient care with members of the allied health professions; and *directing* the family and the nursing auxiliary as they give nursing care—all these affect the goodness of nursing care.

Nursing care is a component of nursing practice that can be divided into two parts: 1) direct nursing care that is performed *with the patient,* and 2) indirect nursing care that is performed away from the patient but *in his behalf.* Most of the latter deals with communication and coordination between nurses and the patient's family, nurses themselves, and members of the medical and allied professions, medical technicians, and management —in industry, schools, hospitals, wherever the patient may be. And these, too, affect the goodness of nursing care and are an integral part of comprehensive nursing care. But in this discussion. I shall limit my concept of good nursing care to that component of nursing practice which is *direct nursing care.*

The word "care" has precise meaning. It belongs to the intellect and its root is in "sorrow." Care *is not akin* to cure. It is more related to "pathos" in that the feelings are touched. When one gives care, the feeling is experienced and responded to by extending oneself toward another. Care is expressed in tending to another, being with him, assisting or protecting him, giving heed to his responses, guarding him from danger that might befall him, providing for his needs and wants with compassion as opposed to sufferance or tolerance; with tenderness and consideration as opposed to a sense of duty; with respect and concern as opposed to indifference.

---

* *Regional Planning for Nursing and Nursing Education.* Report of Work Conference held at Plymouth State Teachers College, Plymouth, New Hampshire, June 12–23, 1950. New York: Bureau of Publications, Teachers College, Columbia University, 1950, p. 8.

Reprinted, with permission, from *Nursing Outlook, V,* 1957, 302–304.

There can be little modification when the word "care" is used in conjunction with the word "nursing"—which has its root in "nourish"—except to enlarge or enrich the meaning. There is some qualification of who is cared for when applied to nursing. Nursing care of the sick, the disabled, the diseased, the disoriented, the disturbed, the infant, the injured, the invalid, the infirm, the handicapped, the helpless, the hopeless, the young, the child, the young mother, the young couple, the old couple, the unwanted, the unwanting, the weak, those who are weary unto death. Margaret Mead stated this qualification with profound simplicity as "the vulnerable" when she said the object of nursing was "to protect the vulnerable."

I have tried to define nursing care as acting and interacting with the patient through physical and personal contact for his welfare, and intervening in his behalf between him and those stresses in the physical environment and in the social climate that impinge upon him. The nursing operations to carry this through I have listed as 1) ministering to the basic human needs, 2) administering medicines, tests, and treatment, 3) observing the patient's response and adaptation, 4) teaching self-care, or counseling on health, 5) supervising or guiding the patient's rehabilitative activities in modifications of daily living, 6) planning with the patient for self-care, which is an outgrowth of managing the care for him—determining and timing the course of action and controlling the manner of its performance, and 7) communicating with the patient throughout all of these—to develop a sense of trust, a feeling of significance and ultimately of self-realization.

The operation that distinguishes nursing care from the care of any other helping profession, is its ministrations—doing for a person that which he would do for himself but is unable to do for a time or for all times; performing these nursing measures of personal and mental hygiene as he would if he were able. The basic ministrations in nursing care are comforting measures that contribute to the sense of well-being—being there and seeing him, bathing, feeding, toileting, dressing, listening to him, moving and sheltering him, and feeling his feelings. To comfort is an object of care. Ministrations are the nursing measures from which all other nursing operations can draw comfort. They are a way and means to establishing mutual trust and confidence—a sense of significance and self-worth. This is fundamental to the "good" performance of all other nursing operations, because all other operations without ministrations do not seem to me to be care— they may be related to cure, but not to care in the meaning of the word.

The administration of medicine, tests or treatments, or assisting with their administration, is a nursing operation that is akin to *cure*. It is also *care* when it is directed to assisting the patient through the experiences, and any assistance given to the doctor, therapist, or technician is subordinate to the care of the patient. Assisting the doctor, rather than the patient, is carrying out a medical technical operation, and not giving *care*.

The administration of medicine, tests, and treatments is the nursing operation that is delegated by medical authority, and the nursing objective parallels and depends upon the medical objective. These nursing operations support the purpose of and implement the therapeutic regimen.

The medical objective may be sustenal, palliative, custodial, or maintenal; the nursing operations necessary to support it may be limited and simple in nature. This is a type of nursing care that can be termed elementary. The medical objective may be remedial, restorative, curative, or controlling of a chronic disease. The nursing operations to support it may be many and complex, and may require knowledge and application of some principles. This type of medical care requires nursing of a technical type, and that is dependent on medical authority.

Consideration of the patient's condition and the patient's capacity and potential, and the existing and potential resources in the situation help to determine the medical objective. Facilities, materials, equipment, organization, philosophy, policies, practices, procedures, and regulations in the agencies; custom, traditions, and mores in the community; availability, competence, organization of personnel, utilization and development of personnel—all these enter into the consideration.

Judgment today dictates that a palliative or maintenal regimen for some patients may be—all things considered—the optimum objective that can be attained at this time.

If the potential of the patient is such, rehabilitizing care is more economical than the sustenal or maintenal. Best judgment today also dictates that prevention, promotion of health, and comprehensive care hold the greatest promise for human progress.

If the medical object is rehabilitative it requires, in addition to those mentioned, three major classifications of nursing operations. The first of these is teaching—personal hygiene, mental hygiene, telling, informing, answering, demonstrating self-care; interpreting regimen, nature of illness, self-observation and testing progress to control; recognition of danger signs and appropriate action of self-care or self-observation, and testing progress and activities; helping in problem solving and teaching groups of patients.

The second is supervision—those exercises that have been prescribed by other therapies, for dietary control, ambulation and elevation, coordination and manipulation, also guiding practice of speech, of bladder and bowel control, other self-care activities that have implications for daily living.

And the third is planning and management—so we move in rehabilitation from management of care in the patient's behalf to planning with him and his family for self-care, for home care, for family care, for use of community resources, for appointments and schedules in the use of these.

This nursing care is a therapeutic type of nursing and it is interdependent, through cooperation and collaboration, with others of the helping professions.

Now, if the medical object extends to comprehensive care, then by definition of the word, it must encompass all of the above, and in addition is an interdisciplinary concern for the patient's continued physical, psychological, and social health and well being. The nursing care is of a comprehensive type only when the nursing is an integral part of this approach.

In comprehensive care the extension of oneself toward another takes on the deeper meaning of "the self" in all nursing operations but communication is the predominant one. Communication extends in a number of directions. First, there is the patient, his feelings about himself, searching for evidence of his strength of motivation, his concern or lack of it, concern about his condition, his relationships, or his life situation, his adaptation or routinization and habituation, his confusions, his spirits, his relationship with family members, his goals, their goals, his present way of meeting problems as they arise. *This is search for a professional estimate of the patient's capacity for adaptation.*

Then there is communicating with allied professional workers such as the social worker and visiting nurse, for their evaluation of the family strength and unity, the role of the patient within it, some estimate of the effect of the change in his role on the family, and which of them might assist with carrying out the regimen or routinization. There is also communication with the psychologist and speech therapist for appraisal of the type of speech involvement, cognition and execution of the practice of speech, the ways of training; and, with the vocational counselor about the possibility of his place in a work situation. There is communication with the doctor, the psychiatrist, the physical or occupational therapist for an estimate of the organic and functional involvement and of the capacity for physical and social rehabilitation. And finally, there is communication with all of these professional workers as they periodically evaluate the patient's care, participating as a contributing member in the evaluation of his progress and assessing the professional care he receives and needs, and with them planning other approaches or steps in his rehabilitation, and planning with the patient also for continuity of nursing care as part of the community health services.

All of this, by way of definition and delineation or description, cannot qualify nursing care as to its goodness. Again this is an attempt to qualify goodness by what goes into nursing care that makes it good.

Nursing is not only the performance of skills and techniques. Nursing care is the care of people, with the responsibility of the nurse to understand people, their motivation and behavior. The use of this understanding throughout all her care of those people she serves to their ultimate well being is an interaction operation, and it must be considered as one index in measuring the goodness of nursing care because it permeates all nursing operation. The criteria of performance, such as safety, comfort, therapeutic effectiveness, the economy of time, effort and materials, the organization, simplicity and adaptivity of planning, and finished workmanship are all affected by the personal interaction.

It is through the use of interaction that the ministrations and observations are aimed at developing the feeling in the patient that he is wanted and that he can trust the nurse. It is through the use of the administration of tests, medicines, and treatments that he is helped to feel significant and that develops confidence in those who serve him. And through the teaching and supervision of his modifications of living he comes to feel self-sufficient and confident that he can rely upon the nurse. With self-management he comes to feel self-reliance and that he has established relationships upon which he can count, not only with the nurse but also with members of the allied professional groups.

My concept of good nursing care is that it is affected by each of the other components of practice, and by the goodness of the supporting functions of teaching, administration, consultation and research; that it is affected by the goodness of medical care only to the extent that it is dependent upon medical authority.

My concept of nursing care is that it differs with the type of care—elementary, technical, therapeutic, or comprehensive, and that the quality of goodness must be measured cumulatively and differently for each of these types. What is good maintenal care may not be good therapeutic care, what is good teaching may be only a part of comprehensive nursing care.

My concept of nursing care is that care is a catalyst that changes nursing operations from technically curative to personal services.

My concept of good nursing care is based on the use of physical ministrations to provide care as a way and means to obtain *intimate understanding and knowledge* of the person and a way and means *to establish mutual trust.* The understanding of a person and the establishment of mutual trust are essential to "goodness." The ministrations and the communications are independent nursing operations through which the goodness of all other operations is affected.

I do not know to what extent this concept of good nursing care is your concept or to what extent it might be commonly accepted by other nurses, by lay people, or allied groups. I do know that I rarely find it, and yet I believe it should be available to people. I know that young women can learn to give it, because I have seen some nurses practice it with great satisfaction. I know it is difficult to do—for I myself keep trying with equal humility. I do believe that it can be provided in the community, but not without some change in the role we play, particularly in hospitals.

I believe that the quality of nursing care we provide the public is a true reflection of our concept of nursing. To the extent that whatever concept of nursing we hold is clear to us, whatever it may be, we will practice and provide it.

22.
A Philosophy of Nursing

by Dorothy Johnson

What is nursing? A philosophical question of a few years ago has become an urgent cry as professional nurses seek to find and establish anew their identity in a rapidly expanding group of health workers. We seemed so sure of ourselves and of our contribution at the turn of the century. Our conceptions of what nursing is are blurred today. Has nursing really changed or have we been diverted from important basic concepts?

In a comparatively few short years, the full flowering of an urban and industrial revolution and a changing pattern of family life have resulted in mushrooming of hospitals and a shift in the locus of the care of the sick from the home to that bureaucratic institution, the hospital. Advances in the natural and behavioral sciences and in medicine and public health have brought to light new knowledge, almost incredible in its amount, scope, and complexity. Numerous new categories of health workers have developed as we attempt to encompass that knowledge and put it to work. Health values and practices of the general public are also changing as these both respond to and influence health programs and services.

The increasing complexity of medical and nursing care has given rise to specialization, fragmentation of the individual and of services, and a division of labor which, in nursing, has opened the door to large numbers of subprofessional and auxiliary nursing personnel. This group, made up of persons of varying levels of training and carrying out specific parts of the total nursing job, has been interspersed between patient and professional nurse. This flowing stream of what are often conflicting social forces has served to diffuse our

Reprinted, with permission, from *Nursing Outlook, VII,* 1959, pp. 198–200.

thoughts and energies and to confuse our goals—in short, it has tended to divide us into at least two camps.

There are those of us who firmly believe that the professional nurse of the future will have largely supervisory and managerial responsibilities and that educational programs should be geared to this end. This view has much to support it since, in reality, there is already a marked trend in this direction in practice. There is also evidence that newly emerging graduates of some schools hold this kind of self-image. The group of nurses who are committed to this camp sometimes find it difficult to admit to this belief, perhaps because it breaks so fundamentally with our history and tradition. In their ambivalence, they say they regret this trend and hold society responsible for those actions which tend to support the movement.

In another camp, there are those of us who believe equally firmly that nursing can and will find its place as a professional discipline only in relation to direct service to people in need of nursing care. Among allied professional groups, certainly, the focus of the majority of practitioners is on service to the individual or to a group of individuals. History, tradition, and the self-image of the majority of nursing practitioners provide powerful support for this view.

There is a major practical problem to be resolved if this view is to regain lost ground and become more widely accepted, however. Nursing care is made up of numerous activities now assumed by several groups of nursing service personnel and is provided within the framework of bureaucratic institutions under delegated and divided responsibility. It is difficult to visualize, under such circumstances, how the professional nurse can develop the kind of responsibility for the care of *her* patients that the physician assumes for *his* patients or the social worker for *her* clients.

The purpose of this paper is not to debate the merits of the views of either camp, but a brief presentation of the issue is essential to understanding the point of view from which it is developed. It is within the context of professional nursing as a direct service to people that some ideas about nursing and its practice are discussed.

The Science of Nursing

The science of nursing, if it exists (I think it does), has yet to be identified. Our concepts of the nature of that science are fuzzy, indeed, but that it is an applied science, as is true of the professions generally, seems fairly certain. Our growing interest in research and our increasing skills in this area, together with some hunches as to the unique nature of nursing, will in time provide an answer to the "if" and, perhaps, the beginnings of a body of knowledge which can be called the science of nursing.

Today, the knowledge we use in nursing care, however adequate or inadequate it may be, concerns primarily the recipient of nursing, the patient, rather than nursing itself, and this imbalance may lead to confusion in establishing nursing goals or developing appropriate plans of nursing action. A knowledge of people and their responses to stress provides the foundation for any health service—for nursing care, for medical care, for social casework—and it is knowledge which we share in common, at least in large measure, with all professional health workers.

Given a particular patient with a particular pattern of response to stress (and this knowledge of people we share in common), each of these professional disciplines offers some unique service, based on a unique body of knowledge within that discipline. What does nursing offer? The answer to this question will form eventually the science of nursing, and the service rendered will be a more soundly based art. Nursing does make a contribution today although what is offered depends upon the individual nurse concerned. Her contribution is largely experientially derived, frequently technical in character, often based on trial and error approaches, and even intuitive in nature. Good, bad, or indifferent, what nursing offers is passed on from nurse to nurse primarily by word of mouth and is sometimes referred to, half facetiously, as "the tricks of the trade."

This kind of information, developed empirically, emphasizes the action required rather than the theoretical foundations of that action. That our contributions have so often been helpful is probably because our experientially derived methods have been tested for many years and the art of nursing, or the service, is identified and communicated more readily than the science.

The chances of today's contribution being effective can be increased even while we await the development of a true science of nursing and the validation of its concepts and theories. We can increase our knowledge and understanding of people: biologically, intrapersonally, interpersonally, and as members of society. We can use that knowledge to sharpen our observations of their requirements for nursing care. We can increase our skills in perception and our ability to think logically, soundly, and searchingly regarding cause and effect to the end that the important factors pertinent to establishing realistic and appropriate objectives in nursing care are considered. We can seek to base our approaches to patients on firmer foundations by clarifying in our own minds what we are trying to do, why, and what scientific knowledge is involved.

We must be more intensively and more definitely concerned with the why, what, and how of making a nursing diagnosis, of developing a plan of nursing care, and of evaluating that care.

The very use of the word diagnosis, even though qualified by the word nursing, may make some of you shudder. It may not be appropriately used, though it does serve the purpose of pointing up the independent judgments and activities required of the professional nurse. If we are correct in our conviction that nursing is a profession, and if our drive for colleague equality in working with the allied professions is soundly motivated, then we must accept the existence of *nursing* problems which require assessment, decision, and action.

These are problems related to, but apart from, medical problems in which we have traditionally shared responsibility through our observations and through delegated authority to administer medications, tests, and treatments. Implicit even within these dependent activities, there is a large area for independent judgment which has not been explicitly recognized or sanctioned. One of our urgent tasks in nursing is to increase our knowledge in ways that will improve our ability to make reasonably valid judgments within the range of nursing practice.

The Art of Nursing

Of all the activities which comprise nursing practice, Frances Kreuter attributes the unique contribution of nursing to its ministrations to the basic human needs of patients. *(Nursing Outlook* May 1957). The various tasks or activities which fall within this component of nursing care—feeding, bathing, toileting, and so forth—are those for which only nursing, of all the professional health disciplines, is responsible. These are the only activities which are not shared in some way with other groups. It is also within this area that a high percentage of *nursing* problems occur. The activities involved in ministering to basic human needs provide our opportunity to carry on the other activities involved in nursing practice and increase the effectiveness of patient care as a whole. It is interesting but a little disturbing to note that these are the very activities which we have delegated first to auxiliary members of the nursing team.

The administrative component of nursing care, on the other hand—a component which is largely delegated and controlled by the physician and which requires primarily technical skills—is clung to zealously and jealously by the professional nurse. This division of labor, which began only a few years ago, is becoming firmly entrenched in nursing practice despite the distinction made almost as soon as modern nursing was born between true nursing care and the following of doctors' orders. Widespread recognition and acceptance of the concept that nursing is more than the carrying out of medical orders has been delayed for many reasons, not the least of which may be the higher status presently accorded those who possess the necessary technical skills to assist the physician in his tasks.

The following advice given to the religious who nursed in the fourteenth century ("Proposal of the Blessed Johannes Ruysbroek") offers a slogan that could become our battle cry:

> Brother, if you are in ecstacy, exalted like St. Peter and St. Paul, or whatever example you wish to take, and you hear that the sick are in need of warm soup or any other assistance, I here give you counsel: leave your meditation immediately and come down to earth and warm the soup.

Any discussion designed to clarify nursing care or to formulate a nursing care plan that I have seen or heard in recent years has emphasized that the human or individual needs of the patient form the basis for care and must be considered. We have not, however, emphasized that ministering to the basic human needs of individuals is the essence, the very heart, of professional nursing.

It may be helpful at this point to look at professional nursing from another perspective. Johnson and Martin in a recent sociological analysis of the nurse role discuss function as the consequence of activities rather than the activities themselves. (*The American Journal of Nursing* March 1958). They attempt to clarify nursing function by looking at "what the nurse is basically doing for the patient," that is, her role and contribution with respect to the maintenance of the social system of doctor-nurse-patient. It is their contention that the primary role of the nurse within this system is to maintain its internal equilibrium through managing the tensions which arise among the system members.

We have given credence to this point of view for many years as we have talked about the nurse as the liaison between doctor and patient, and more recently have come to use the more sophisticated term, "therapeutic environment." Johnson and Martin point out that the patient's tensions, generated as a result of illness or growing out of activities designed to get him well, tend to be reduced or released as the nurse makes explanations, offers reassurance, and provides comforting ministrations which are immediately gratifying to the patient. Such reduction in tension allows available energy then to be concentrated on activities which assist in diagnosis or treatment and thus contributes to the doctor's primary function of getting the patient well.

This concept of the nurse role offers dignity to the ministrative component of nursing care. The ministrations provide the medium through which the role is played out and the function is made possible. Such concepts provide an exciting theoretical frame of reference for research into the science of nursing. They enrich our ideas of nursing—what it is and what it is not. If we accept this concept, our activities must inevitably be person-centered rather than task-centered, and our notions of desirable approaches to patients in solving nursing problems become subject to study in relation to their specific contribution to patient welfare.

The concept proposed by Johnson and Martin also serves to clarify a difference between the doctor role and the nurse role of vital importance to present and future relationships between members of the two professions. We have tended to be rather critical of physicians who have partially or completely failed to play a role which Johnson and Martin perceive as primarily the nurse role, that is, to provide suitable outlets for tensions and to offer immediate gratifications in response to expressed need. If these investigators are right in their contention that the physician cannot give primacy to both roles and must be concerned with getting the patient well, then our criticism is not only unjustified and unrealistic but actually detrimental to patient welfare.

Physicians, on the other hand, have been equally critical of us, feeling that we have not given proper attention to the technical aspects of getting the patient well and have been too involved in his emotional reactions. It does behoove us to give adequate consideration to technical procedures, but for the purpose of delegation to auxiliary members of the nursing team. As Mary Kelly Mullane has pointed out recently: "Maintaining the personal, spiritual support of patients may well require that professional nurses reduce to routine tasks as many technical procedures as they can, and then delegate them to nursing assistants. Otherwise, professional nurses will be so occupied with the routines of treatments, medications, and checking charts, that the heart of nursing, indeed the heart of medical care, will be lost completely." (*Nursing Outlook* June 1958).

If we can visualize a clear-cut division of labor in which each discipline has a primary and specific contribution to patient welfare and only a secondary contribution which is related to the primary contribution of the other, and if this concept is recognized and sanctioned by both medicine and nursing, our effectiveness as a team would be enhanced immeasurably. Our conflicts and misunderstanding have all too often left the patient alone in the middle of this three-way system, progressing haltingly, if at all, toward recovery.

The Common Core in Nursing

Thus far, I have been discussing nursing as an entity. This entire article has been developed on the premise that there is a common core in nursing—

in its science and in its art—and that practitioners of nursing use that core in many settings, with varying age groups, and at various levels of employment. This common core has almost been lost from sight in our increasing trend toward specialization. It is essential that this core be further developed, tested, and refined, if the discipline of nursing is to advance. Specialization and specialists do have a contribution to make to the science of nursing as a whole, and, as in other professions, to its several parts. Since the science of nursing must develop from attempts to assist people under stress, then it follows that concentrations of people—of different ages and with differing health problems in certain settings—will allow for more intensive study of the related nursing problems as well as the development of the required nursing skills. We must study these problems for their contribution to the core—for the inherent value of such knowledge in nursing care of an individual of a different age, sex, or with an ostensibly different problem. With such a viewpoint, we cease to compete with each other; rather we look for generalizations of knowledge, while at the same time we recognize that some knowledge will be applicable only in specific settings or situations.

What is nursing? It is professional discipline and, as such, a social service. It provides a direct service to individuals—a service which offers comfort, gratification, and assistance at those times when individuals are under stress, and in relation to their basic human needs. In so doing, it further offers an indirect service which makes a specific contribution to the promotion and maintenance of health and to recovery from illness. It involves the ability to assess situations, arrive at decisions, and implement a course of action designed to resolve nursing problems. It has a two-pronged base in knowledge: one, a knowledge of the predictable patterns of behavior of people under stress within a broad category of variables; and, two, a knowledge of the nursing behavior indicated for helpful intervention.

In essence, as Lyle Saunders has put it so beautifully: "Whenever and wherever the nursing function is performed, there are always present two indispensable components, the patient and the nurse—one needing, one giving." (*The American Journal of Nursing* July 1958).

23.

Some Problems in Nursing Care and Services

by Laurie M. Gunter

One significant trend in nursing is the decline in value of nursing care in comparison to the increased value of medical care. Before World War II and the wide use of sulfa drugs, antibiotics, tranquilizers and the phenomenal development of medical research, nurses had about as much to offer the patient as did the physician. For example, the child with typhoid fever needed a nurse in constant attendance to sponge his head, give him nourishment teaspoon by teaspoon, turn him from side to side, bathe and rub his back, promote his desire to live through his suffering, and keep him mindful in subtle ways that life was worth living. The physician could only look at him and give him medicine which probably was not helpful, and certainly not specific for his condition.

As medical research and science have advanced they have enhanced tremendously the contribution of the physician, who in turn has become even more competent and his services more valued by the patient. Evidence of relief or cure of a disease is frequently dramatic, and there are promises of more miracles to come. In comparison, the nurse today is seldom a private duty nurse whom the patient has known and lived with through weeks and months of illness. In fact, the duration of the patient's illness has been drastically reduced and the care he receives during this time is provided by a large variety of personnel. The patient seldom remembers a nurse as *his* nurse, although he knows his physician. In addition, the tranquilizing drugs reduce the patient's anxiety and thus his need for care. Many patients can now manage their own care with only some nursing service.

It is expected that hospitalization periods will be further shortened and may even become virtually nonexistent in the future. Increasingly, medical care will be administered on an outpatient basis.

Thus it seems to me that nursing care has declined in value and is heading toward obsolescence. In addition to the development of medical care, other factors have contributed to this decline. One such factor is the value of activity in this society, as described by Talcott Parsons. Emphasis in health care is now on the patient's return to gainful activity as soon as possible. Dependency, as fostered by the kind of care given before World War II, is actively discouraged and early ambulation is desirable. At one time, mothers, after childbirth, were required to remain in bed from 10 to 14

From an unpublished paper, "Nursing—Some Notes on the Problems and Issues," 1966.

days, during which time they were given care. Today, a new mother is expected and encouraged to assume full responsibility for herself and for her infant within a matter of hours, and she is usually discharged from the hospital within three days.

Another major change that has occurred in nursing during the past twenty years is the elimination of some aspects of nursing care from the domain of nursing service and their assignment to other departments of the hospital. In some of the large teaching medical centers, some specialized nursing care, such as that required by patients undergoing kidney dialysis, and individual nursing care required by some patients are provided through a separate budget; or the costs may be absorbed by medical budgets. In some instances, the decision to provide this type of nursing care is not made by the department of nursing service but by medical staff. Significantly, seriously ill or unconscious patients are placed in "intensive care" units. "Intensive care" is thus distinguished from "nursing care." It provides services to groups of patients, and more efficient use of skilled medical and nursing personnel, costly equipment and medical technologies. The focus is on the diagnostic and therapeutic services to the patient rather than on the promotion of his comfort and well-being, which is characteristic of "nursing care." Furthermore, in the intensive care unit the proportion of the nurse's functions is relatively high, and she works under close medical supervision, functioning largely as an assistant to the physician.

One of the reasons for misunderstanding between nursing service and nursing education is the failure of some nursing educators to distinguish nursing *care* from nursing service. Although it is acknowledged that a registered nurse needs preparation to give nursing *care,* educators seem to be reluctant to face the fact that nurses also need preparation to *organize* nursing care and related activities, the task of nursing service. Nursing care is not required by all patients, and in the interest of economy it should be provided only when needed. However, many leaders in nursing received their preparation at a time when nursing care was an important component of nursing service, and they are now trying to prepare students for activities which were highly valued twenty or thirty years ago but which are less useful for both the patient and the physician today. Nursing education, which at present aims at splitting the registered nurse functions into so-called "professional" and "technical", i.e., separating the interpersonal and communicative skills from the manual and medical assistance skills, and makes separate individuals responsible for each of these activities, does not seem to be providing a logical solution to the problems in nursing. The belief that one can perform manual and medical tasks for a patient without realizing that these are best accomplished through an effective interpersonal relationship, may harm the effectiveness of the so-called "technical nurse." All nurses need skills in human relations. Simply because medicine has become a highly developed technology does not mean that it need become de-humanized.

Monitoring devices and computers will require some skilled technicians in nursing services who may or may not be prepared in schools of nursing. Given the present distinction between nurses in nursing education and those in nursing services, it is highly unlikely that nursing educators have the kind of training and insights they need to keep up with technical developments in hospitals and medicine in general. Collegiate nursing education, in its drive to become "academic" may be in danger of becoming removed from immediate reality, in that it is not practical enough or too speculative. There is current emphasis on conceptualizing and synthesizing theoretical knowledge from the social and natural scientific disciplines without first subjecting these concepts to empirical study in nursing.

In schools of nursing in this country, dividing and limiting the days allotted for clinical experience, coupled with the patient's shortened hospital stay, minimize the student's opportunity for developing a significant interpersonal relationship with the patient. On the other hand, this type of relationship is less necessary for the patient's welfare today. He is admitted to the hospital and participates in such an intensive medical regime that there is little opportunity for him to become known to the nurse or for him to get to know her. Neither does such a plan for clinical experience allow the student to develop expertness in nursing skills and a sense of nursing competence prior to her assumption of responsibility as a registered nurse.

Nursing education, organized to fit the academic structure of the college or university, using the hospital *as if* it were a laboratory, and lacking provision for experience in the real work situation, does not aid in the development of a sense of commitment that is required of the nurse who will assume continuous patient responsibility. Thus the student never realizes the nature of this responsibility, which continues to exist through week-ends and holidays, as clearly as a medical intern or resident does. As a result, many directors of nursing services and hospital administrators consider collegiate nursing programs to be more theoretical than functional.

My predictions for the future include developments in medicine which will further reduce the incidence of disease and the refinement and simplification of medical treatment to the extent of possibly eliminating hospital care. As we can visualize the disappearance of war, we might well foresee the disappearance of disease. Until we arrive at this stage of development, however, we must plan to meet the nursing needs of society, and prepare nurses to function with some satisfaction in the performance of their work.

We can begin by giving our attention to the preparation of registered nurses for the specialized functions required by a highly developed medical technology. The diploma program has traditionally prepared for the registered nurse functions. Relatively recently the four- to five-year collegiate programs have evolved from this traditional type of program and even more recently the two-year collegiate programs have developed. These various types of programs all prepare for nurse registration.

It would seem urgent that university schools of nursing, which have teaching medical center hospitals available, utilize their rich and varied resources by providing academic programs leading to higher degrees and certification programs for nurse specialists, so that nurses may function at a level above that of registered nurse. Three general areas of preparation appear to be necessary at this stage. They are: the management of nursing care and services; nursing specialization; and teaching and research. At the present time, many masters programs in nursing are trying to achieve a composite preparation in clinical specialization, introductory research, and teaching, supervision or administration. Can masters preparation encompass these broad areas within one program of study at more than a superficial or introductory level?

Given the dearth of faculty with preparation for university teaching and research, it would seem expedient to discontinue what appears in many schools to be the isolation from academic departments and professional schools. Programs should be developed in collaboration with these in order to utilize appropriately scholars in the university, and so that nurses may assume responsibilities comparable to other scholars and professionals.

Unless a different kind of preparation is offered to nurses for the management functions in nursing services, these will be performed by individuals who have been trained in other disciplines. At the present time adequate preparation of this kind is not included in the basic nursing program. Collaboration with schools of business might provide nurses with the kind of knowledge that would provide the basis for the achievement of a level of excellence in nursing services rarely seen today.

It is true that attention has been given to the preparation of teachers for schools of nursing. But with the current emphasis on clinical specialization within these programs at the masters level, we may do well to question how much preparation for teaching is really given in these programs, whether this kind of preparation is necessary, and if so, is it possible that it could best be obtained in collaboration with schools of education where current research is leading to the development of effective methods and technologies. Preparation for nurses in basic science disciplines is already being supported by the United States Public Health Service under the Nurse Scientist Programs and Special Nurse Fellowships. Nurses with this preparation may apply this knowledge to nursing practice and use it to develop research methods needed in nursing. They will have preparation for university teaching and research.

Even less attention has been given to thoughtful consideration of the preparation of nursing specialists. For one thing, this type of preparation does not lend itself to the academic course structure of the university. Long hours of experience and practice in the hospital setting are needed to develop specialized skills and clinical judgment. Planned experience of a kind similar to that which is used for the preparation of medical specialists may have value in the preparation of nursing specialists. The development of these kinds of programs could be facilitated by collaboration with schools of medicine. If nursing is not willing to prepare some nurses for medical assistant functions through nursing specialization, then other workers will be trained to do the job. Thus nursing may become arrested at the level of the registered nurse unless more adequate and realistic preparation is provided for the functions of management of nursing services and nursing specialization.

Essential to the survival of nursing in a rapidly changing social order is a realistic appraisal of where we are in nursing education and practice, a realistic consideration of whether there is need for change and, if so, in what direction, and the development of valid and reliable methods of appraisal of consequences of actions, rather than verbal claims to professional status and grandiose accomplishments. That nursing is a profession, that the baccalaureate program in nursing prepares for professional practice, that the placement of nursing education in institutions for higher education will solve the socio-economic status problems and prestige needs of nurses may be myths which are in process of colliding with reality.

24.

Tenderness and Technique: Nursing Values in Transition

by Genevieve Rogge Meyer

This research has been a study of nursing values in transition, and its organizing theme has been the fluctuating relationship between the two major nursing traditions of *tenderness* and *technique*. In terms of our historical interpretation, the startling changes in nursing brought about during the last

Los Angeles: Institute of Industrial Relations, University of California at Los Angeles, 1960, pp. 113–117.

half of the nineteenth century by the persevering efforts of Florence Nightingale included the raising of both moral and technical standards for nursing. To use her words, nurses had to have both character and knowledge. Thus, in her program tenderness and technique were contained in a balanced and integrated relationship. Both were essential to sound nursing practice.

Then in the early part of the twentieth century, at least in the United States, the balanced relationship between tenderness and technique began to shift and the technical tradition gained greater prominence. (The first schools based on the Nightingale system had been started in this country in 1873.) This shift represented a response to the demands of rapidly developing medical technology during the 1920's and 1930's, though it had earlier origins perhaps in the general emphasis on more scientific business and industrial organization that characterized this country in the years surrounding World War I. Nurses found themselves involved in more technical procedures, and the value placed on tenderness receded somewhat as the image of the efficient, coolly controlled practitioner gained prestige. Apparently the depression also played a role in this transition as nurses began to learn that altruistic tenderness did not in itself bring economic security.

But the very need for nurses to take on an expanding number of technical functions created another sort of need. Someone had to take over the simpler tasks that nurses no longer had time for; and other workers began to be added to the roster of nursing service personnel—first the aide, and later the trained practical nurse. This added still other duties, of an administrative and supervisory character, to the nurse's load; as a result, the technical role has actually grown into the administrative-technical role.

How these added administrative and supervisory responsibilities affected the nurse's typical work situation was the first question explored by the research. According to our sample of R.N.'s, the work situation that was most typical of nursing 20 years ago consisted of the nurse working alone with her patient. This was followed by the nurse working with her patient plus a colleague—either a doctor or another nurse. The nurse at work just with her colleague was felt to have been least typical. Today, however, the situation believed to be most typical consisted of the nurse working with a colleague, whereas the nurse alone with her patient was considered least typical. The sharing work relationship was again in the middle. Attitudes toward these changes—measured in terms of personal preferences for the three types of work situations—were varied. Some nurses preferred the work situation typical of nursing 20 years ago, some liked the situation typical today, and two other groups preferred the sharing work relationship.

This introduced the main part of the research. Four types of nurses were defined on the basis of their responses to the Nursing Picture Item Test, and these four value types were conceived as representing different adaptations to the fluctuating relationship between the two value traditions of tenderness and technique. Type I (ministering angel) preferred an unshared relationship with her patient and was interpreted as representing the nurse who places a higher value on tenderness than on technique. Type IV (efficient, disciplined professional), on the other hand, preferred to work in an exclusive relationship with her colleague, and her orientation was interpreted as a valuation of technique over tenderness. As it turned out, Type I preferred the ways of yesterday while Type IV liked the work situations typical of nursing today. The other two groups were the modern Types II and III who solved the potential conflict between patient and colleague, between tenderness and technical-administrative values, by integrating them, that is, by preferring to work in a situation which included the nurse, her patient, and her colleague too. The two modern groups were differentiated by the fact that Type II was drawn into the sharing situation more by the patient, while Type III was more attracted by the colleague. In this sense Type II's solution was closer to the dominant orientation of Type I, while Type III was closer to Type IV.

The integrations that seem to be happening in the case of Types II and III indicate that a new relationship between tenderness and technique is, and has been, in the making. It has been suggested at several points in this report that the new balance between tenderness and technique has been facilitated, if not prompted, by a move "outward" in nursing, as distinct from the move "upward" to more complex technical functions. The move "outward" has involved a growing concern with 1) the *full* problem of health, including its maintenance as well as its restoration, and 2) the psychological aspects of illness. This has meant the application of the scientific as well as the intuitive method to the problems of supportive emotional care and patient education. To advance these ends the nursing profession has been making use of knowledge from the social sciences, in addition to already accepted knowledge from the biological sciences. This development is making tenderness as worthy as technique. Furthermore, at least in the writer's opinion, the new trend augurs well for the satisfaction of the desire to care for the patient, which, as this research has shown, continues to draw women into nursing.

IV   ECONOMIC PROBLEMS OF THE PROFESSION

Nurses during the first part of the twentieth century were essentially individual practitioners with a one-to-one, face-to-face relationship with their patients. Often a nurse stayed with the same patient for weeks or months at a time, and it was not unusual for a nurse to be called by a family time and time again as different medical crises developed. Under these conditions nurses worked long hours at low wages under hazardous conditions, but they were not particularly concerned with changing the economic basis of their profession. Nurses argued and even believed that since the sick were not conscious of the hours or days, it would be unprofessional for the nurse to be concerned about hours and pay. Moreover they felt that by limiting the hours of the work week, a nurse would be thrown into the same class as a factory worker. As a result, when the California legislature in 1913 enacted a law regulating the hours of work for women, registered nurses were specifically excluded by their own request.

Even as late as 1926 some 18 percent of private duty nurses worked a twenty-four hour day, and 80 percent worked at least a twelve-hour day. The hourly pay was about 50 cents, the same that the average charwoman was then making. The charwoman, moreover, was assured of more regular employment. Nursing registries did try to set minimum wage standards, but since the registered nurse had to compete with the practical nurse for most cases, the registries dared not raise their standards much. Many nurses were fearful that if salaries were raised and work hours shortened, the net result would be a longer wait between cases, and that would cost them more than they would gain. Nursing organizations therefore tended to concentrate on upgrading education, setting minimum standards for nursing registries, gaining state licensure, and other important tasks, but usually ignored the basic economic questions facing nurses. This silence was broken when the Committee on the Grading of Nursing Schools issued its report. Originally, the mission of the committee had been a dual (and contradictory) one: to raise the standards in

159

nursing schools and yet increase the supply of nurses in order to alleviate what was believed to be a nursing shortage. To find the extent of the nursing shortage the committee began an intensive study, but the members found, to their surprise, that there was a surplus of nurses rather than a shortage. The report of the committee set nurses to thinking about how to better their economic status.

25.
Facing the Economic Facts

by May Ayres Burgess

There seems no question that, at the time this text is being written (March, 1928) employment conditions for private duty nurses are extremely bad. The American Journal of Nursing reports that for some time past notices have been received for insertion in its pages from official district registries saying in effect, "We do not wish to seem inhospitable, but employment conditions in this region are so poor that we urge upon nurses in other cities to investigate before coming here." These conditions are not confined to one or two sections of the country, but seem to be rather general.

Two questions were asked concerning present employment conditions which at first seemed to have resulted in mutually contradictory answers. The first was: "Is your registry receiving more or less calls now than it did a year ago?"; and the second: "Are present employment conditions better or worse than they were a year ago?"

Of all the registries combined, 56 percent said that they were receiving fewer calls; while at the same time 63 percent said that conditions were either the same, or better.

An analysis of the returns, however, showed that the returns from hospital registries were markedly different, in each case, from those of the other sorts of registries. Some 54 percent of hospital registries are getting as many or more calls, but only 28 percent of the other registries. Similarly 20 percent of the hospital registries say that present conditions are definitely better, as compared with 13 percent of the other registries.

The picture apparently is something like this. Hospital registries are getting more calls, either because they have more patients, or because the patients are willing to pay for special nurses as they were not a few years ago. To the

From *Nurses, Patients and Pocketbooks*. New York: Committee on the Grading of Nursing Schools, 1928, pp. 83–85, 427–433.

head of a hospital registry, employment conditions are "good" if the hospital can get enough nurses (preferably from among its own alumnae) to meet its own demands for specials and if its own alumnae are reasonably well employed. As the number of its own alumnae grows, the hospital naturally does not have to call upon the outside registries, and accordingly the business of these registries drops.

For many of the outside registries, the fact that the hospitals are now meeting their own nursing needs from their own alumnae, has meant a serious drop in business. For these registries last year there was a real unemployment problem. For the coming year there will, apparently, be a worse one.

The figures indicate that conditions are becoming especially serious in the large cities. In cities of 500,000 or over only 9 percent of the hospital registries, and 3 percent of the outside registries report that conditions are "better," whereas 43 percent of the hospital registries and 68 percent of the outside registries report that they are definitely worse. The ideal state from the hospital viewpoint would probably be one in which the hospital had so many alumnae that it never had to go outside for its supply of specials; and yet did not have so many alumnae that it could not provide employment for all of them within its own walls. So long as the hospital remains in this ideal middle ground, employment conditions will be "good," but, if either it has too few, or too many alumnae, conditions become unsatisfactory. The returns seem to indicate that many hospitals in the largest cities have reached or are close to reaching the third stage where they are unable to offer adequate employment to large numbers of their own graduates.

The following comment from the superintendent of a large metropolitan hospital illustrates what is happening.

In 1925 and 1926 we had a yearly average of practically 7,000 calls. About 4,300 of these calls were covered by our own graduates, but about 2,000 calls went to nurses in outside registries, and another 700 went unfilled. We usually had a daily average of 250 nurses enrolled.

In 1927, however, although we had practically the same number of calls (nearly 7,000) we were able to fill well over 6,000 of them from our own alumnae. We employed only 734 outside nurses, and had only 34 calls unfilled. One of the reasons for this change was that by 1927 the daily average of nurses enrolled on our registry had increased from 250 to 329.

Knowing that this hospital graduates in the neighborhood of 80 new nurses a year, one wonders how long it will be before its supply of alumnae becomes an embarrassment of riches! Yet the figures gathered by the Grading Committee strongly suggest that something like this situation is already developing in many different schools.

● ● ●

Nursing is an idealistic profession, but that fact does not render it immune to economic considerations. Except in the Sisterhoods, the Spirit of Nursing is in perpetual conflict with the economic fact; and whenever economic conditions in nursing begin to be unhealthy, it is the damage to the Spirit of Nursing which shows first evidences that something is wrong. If nurses are intelligent in their desire to maintain the best of what nursing stands for, they will probably do well to make a careful study of the laws of supply and demand which apply not only to nursing, but to other professions as well.

One of these laws may be stated as follows: *Under healthful conditions the number of workers in a profession bears a close relation to the amount of adequately paid work available for them.* In other words, there is no civic virtue in enticing hundreds of new recruits into a profession unless there is some work in sight at which they can earn a living after they get in. It is not enough to say, "Humanity needs them!" Wages in the United States are good, the standard of living is high, what the public wants it rather adequately manages to get. If humanity wants nursing, it will pay for it, just as it pays for automobiles; and if it does not want nursing, it will not buy it. Therefore, it would seem wise (unless some definite promises can be secured for ample and long term subsidies) for the nursing and medical professions to begin at once an energetic inquiry not merely into "How much nursing would it be good for people to have?" but "How much and what sorts of nursing is the public ready to buy?"

More than a quarter of a century ago the medical profession began to make a careful study of its field. Perhaps unconsciously, but directly as the result of its efforts to improve the quality of its graduates, it reduced the number of colleges by half. It is still actively and conscientiously employed in limiting new recruits to the profession to young men and women of high quality in sufficient numbers to provide adequate medical care for the expected population at each decade, but not to result in a flooding of the medical market. Is it reasonable to suggest that nursing might well follow the same policy?

At the present time there are apparently three nurses to every two physicians in the United States. Except in some rural districts and in a few specialties, physicians almost unanimously report that there is no shortage of nurses in their localities. The typical physician reporting in this study had, on the day he answered the questionnaire, three patients who needed special nurses and two who got them; but the third patient was not the victim of a nursing shortage. According to medical testimony, the third patient went without a nurse because he did not want her enough to pay her price. The physicians who provided the material which has gone into this study are a selected group. They represent that part of the medical profession which is particularly interested in nursing problems, and that means the part which most frequently has occasion to employ special duty nurses. If in this report the average physician had only three patients who needed special nursing care and only two who were willing to buy it, it seems reasonable to believe that the average for the whole profession would be even lower.

Registries for private duty nurses report serious country-wide unemployment. Physicians report an ample supply of nurses. Yet there are only three nurses to every two physicians at the present time. What then is going to happen in 1965 when, according to the extremely conservative estimates, there will apparently be nine or ten nurses for every two physicians?* Can the physicians treble their use of special nurses and persuade their patients to pay the cost?

More than half the nurses are in private duty. If there were some obvious opening for nurses in one of the other fields, might the increased production be taken care of? Here, perhaps, is the real answer to part of the problem, but it needs qualification. Every one is agreed that there is need for more public health nursing; yet, . . . for every public health nursing position filled in the month of March, 1927, there were five applicants. There is no shortage of applicants for public health nursing. There is a lack of applicants properly prepared to do public health work, but the shortage is one of quality, not quantity. Moreover, even in this field there is real question of how many new workers can be absorbed. Public health salaries are low as it is. Public health nurses, so far as one can judge, are apt to hold on to their positions rather tenaciously, and do not step aside to make room for newcomers.

No estimates are available at present, but it would seem rather important that the nursing profession attempt some evaluation not only of how much public health nursing the country might beneficially receive, but of how many new nursing positions *with salaries attached* are likely to be created each year. Is the public so eager for public health nursing that it will buy more of it and at the same time not try to cut down on the amount of money it is spending for salaries for the present workers? Until the nursing profession has some answer to this question, how can it tell whether or not it should be seeking many thousands of new workers? Five applicants for every position, even though they be poorly trained, must, it would seem, inevitably have some effect upon keeping present salaries perilously near the minimum level, below which self-respecting professional women will decide that they cannot afford to go.

In institutional work there would appear to be a definite shortage, but is it one which can be looked upon as the solution for disposing of the horde of new workers? Apparently, almost all hospitals are seriously understaffed.

---

* Ed. note: Most recent available figures at this printing indicate a little more than 4 nurses for every 2 physicians as of January 1964.

Many of them have no graduate nurses at all for the care of their patients. Here, one would say, is the great untilled field for nursing. Perhaps it may be. If the nursing profession can persuade hospital authorities that the trained nurse is better for the care of patients than either the student or the attendant, there perhaps may be the solution of where the 60,000 graduates of 1965 can go.*

The estimates given . . . are conservative. . . . the logarithmic curve used . . . to predict the numbers of graduates each year in the future might, with almost equal fairness, have been so calculated on the basis of the existing data that the annual crops of graduates in the future would be much larger than the estimates given. Instead of a graduating class in 1965 of 60,000, the estimate might perhaps, with equal validity, have been for 80,000 or 90,000.

Moreover, the computations of total nurses actively engaged in the profession for each year in the future have been based upon records supplied by superintendents of nurses for past graduates of their schools. It is known that these records have failed to include reports for large numbers of married graduates who have left the profession only to return later. It seems to be a phenomenon of American life, not peculiar to the nursing profession but to be seen in every field, that married women are increasingly keeping on with their professional activities. It is impossible at present to estimate how great this tendency now is or how rapidly it will continue to grow, but it seems safe to say that the numbers of nurses in active practice each year in the future would be enlarged considerably over the estimates . . . if it were possible to predict how many of the married nurses will each year return to active professional practice. They would be even more increased if estimates were included covering nurses coming into the United States from other countries.

It is not desired to exaggerate conditions, but it is believed that there is at hand ample warrant for calling attention to the possibility of serious overproduction in the nursing profession and raising the question which must be faced: "How are we going to provide adequate paid employment for nurse graduates?"

* Ed. note: The graduating class of the academic year 1963–1964 numbered 35,260.

The Burgess Report had indicated that hospitals might serve as a growing source of employment for nurses, and in this the report proved prophetic. The University of Chicago Hospitals began, about the time of the report, to rely entirely on graduate nurses for staffing, and the trend, once started, gained momentum nationally. The growth in the number of hospital nurses was accelerated during the 1930's by unemployment among nurses, improvement in aseptic techniques, development of new drugs, new equipment, and the changing demands for nursing care. The speed of this transition was increased during World War II by the widespread use of army hospitals and by the development of hospital insurance. By 1945, nursing was no longer a profession that had a one-to-one relationship between nurse and patient; instead, the patient was now just one of many the hospital nurse had to deal with. Unfortunately, the transition was so rapid and so radical, that nurses and nursing groups fell even further behind other groups in their income and economic well being. Furthermore, while nursing had started out as perhaps the only profession for women, it now had to face competition with a wide number of occupations open to women, and it was slow to meet this challenge. This was most evident from a survey made by the U.S. Department of Labor in 1946-47.

26.
The Economic Status of Registered Professional Nurses 1946-47

Earnings and expenses. The average nurse, excluding those living in hospitals, earned about $175 during the month of October 1946—about $1 an hour. These earnings were supplemented by an average of about one meal daily. About one nurse in eight, including about one-fifth of the institutional nurses, lived in hospital quarters; inclusion of the cash earnings of these nurses would not substantially affect the over-all average earnings just quoted. Out of her salary the average nurse spent about $7 a month—$83 annually—on professional expenses in 1946.

The highest monthly earnings were those of nurse educators, who averaged $207 in cash in October 1946. Industrial nurses ranked next, followed by

From Bulletin No. 931, Department of Labor, Bureau of Labor Statistics, Washington, D.C.: U.S. Government Printing Office, 1947, 1–3, 51–53.

public health, institutional, and office nurses. The lowest earnings were those of private duty nurses, who averaged $153 in the month studied. Because of variations in hours worked the rank of these six major fields was different with respect to average hourly earnings. Institutional nurses, the largest group in the profession, had the lowest hourly earnings—87 cents for those providing their own living quarters—although they most frequently received meals in addition to their salary. Industrial nurses stood highest in hourly earnings, with an average of $1.11.

Hours. The typical scheduled workday in nursing is 8 hours. Hours actually worked during October 1946 averaged about 44 a week; about one nurse out of four was on duty for 50 hours or more weekly. Overtime is frequent and typically is not paid for; where it is paid for, compensation is generally in the form of time off rather than any additional cash salary.

The longest hours were reported by institutional nurses, who were on duty an average of 48 hours a week in October 1946, and the shortest hours were those of private duty nurses, who averaged 39 hours weekly. In all fields except institutional work scheduled workweeks of 44 hours or less are typical, and in public health work weekly schedules of 40 hours or less are most common.

In addition to her hours on duty, about one hospital nurse in four was required to be on call, and a corresponding proportion worked split shifts. For those subject to call, time on call amounted to roughly 35 hours a month beyond hours on duty in October 1946.

Most nurses normally work only on the day shift; those on duty at night usually receive the same hourly rate as for day work. Rotation between early and late shifts is slightly more common than continued employment on late shifts.

Vacations, sick leave, and insurance. Except for those on private duty, almost all nurses received paid vacations and four out of five were covered by formal sick leave plans. Vacations were typically 2 weeks long, although 4-week vacations were frequent in institutional and public health work and in nursing education.

Outside the industrial and office fields, most nurses were not covered by retirement pension plans. Nor did nurses typically receive free hospitalization, medical care, or insurance, although these benefits were more common in institutional work than in other branches of the profession.

Variations in working conditions among nursing fields. Working conditions varied appreciably among the six major fields of nursing:

1. Institutional nurses had the lowest hourly pay and the longest hours on duty, but because of their relatively long hours their monthly earnings were above those of both private duty and office nurses. Allowance for meals

received would about equalize the monthly but not the hourly pay of institutional and public health nurses. A substantial minority worked split shifts and had to be on call for some hours beyond their time on duty. Night work was more common in this than in any other field except private duty. Vacation and sick leave provisions were relatively liberal.

2. Nurse educators received the highest monthly earnings of any branch of the profession and had the longest vacations. Although they worked slightly shorter hours than did institutional nurses (with whom they shared many working conditions) their workweek exceeded those in other branches of the profession. While most nurse educators lived outside, they were required to live in hospital quarters more frequently than any other nurses.

3. Because part-time work of some private duty nurses reduced their average hours below those in any other branch, their average monthly earnings in October 1946 were the lowest in any branch of nursing. Their typical hourly rate was, however, exceeded only by the hourly earnings of public health and industrial nurses. Frequently they received one meal daily in addition to their cash salaries. Since private duty nurses continually change employers and are not covered by the Social Security Act, they do not benefit from either private or publicly operated retirement pension plans, vacation and sick leave plans, or medical care arrangements.

4. Of the six branches of nursing, public health nursing ranks second highest in terms of hourly earnings and third in monthly earnings; these earnings are seldom supplemented by meals or laundry of uniforms. Monthly hours on duty are shorter than in any other branch of nursing except private duty. Retirement provisions are relatively more common than in most other branches of nursing, although less than half the public health nurses reported such arrangements. Sick leave was widespread; but public health nurses fared relatively poorly in provisions for medical care and hospitalization.

5. Industrial nurses had the highest hourly earnings. However, their monthly pay was exceeded by that of nurse educators since they worked comparatively short hours. Unlike other nurses, they are protected by both old-age and unemployment compensation provisions of the Social Security Act. Overtime pay and premium pay for night work were most common in this field. Together with office nurses, they received relatively short vacations.

6. Office nurses' monthly pay was the lowest in October 1946 of any field except private duty, and their hourly pay was the lowest except for institutional nurses. Working hours in this field were exceeded by those of institutional nurses and nurse educators; and office nurses were seldom paid in any way for overtime. Formal sick leave arrangements were less frequent than for other nurses.

Regional variations in working conditions. On a regional basis, the best salaries and working conditions, particularly in institutional and private duty work, were found on the Pacific Coast. However, vacations were shorter in these States than elsewhere.

New England ranked lowest in terms of salaries. Split shifts and hours on call were also relatively common in New England, and the proportion of time spent on nonprofessional duties was higher in this region and in the Middle Atlantic States than in the rest of the country. In contrast, New England and Middle Atlantic nurses reported the longest vacations.

Except for New England and the Pacific States, generalization with respect to the relative position of each region is difficult. No one region consistently had the longest hours in all fields in October 1946 (although the Middle West and Southwest tended to have relatively long hours).

Duties. How was the time of the limited number of professional nurses who were active in their profession allocated among different duties? About 30 percent of the "average" hospital nurse's time was spent in making beds, answering lights, carrying trays, bathing and feeding patients, giving back rubs, taking patients to appointments, checking linens and household supplies, and on clerical work (other than nurses' notes). About half of her time was spent on preparing and giving medication, changing dressings, giving aseptic treatments and similar duties, assisting in operations and deliveries, and in supervising other nurses and nonprofessional help. The rest of the day was devoted to a variety of other duties.

• • •

Comparison With Earnings and Working Conditions in Other Fields

In order to provide a background against which the information on earnings and working conditions of registered professional nurses could be evaluated, the Bureau of Labor Statistics attempted to compile available information on earnings in other fields that compete either directly or indirectly with nursing. Two types of information have been assembled here: 1) Data on earnings and working conditions in occupations into which potential nursing students can go without training comparable to that required of registered professional nurses, and 2) earnings and working conditions in occupations and professions employing large numbers of women with a considerable amount of specialized education. Unfortunately, however, the amount of reasonably current information that is available on professional groups in which substantial numbers of women are employed has proved to be very meager.

Earnings. The available information on nonprofessional jobs indicates that while there are many workers in the country earning less than the average nurse, there are occupations requiring much less training that provide hourly pay equal to or above that of most nurses. Thus in October 1946 women assemblers requiring little special training averaged $1 an hour (the average earnings of nurses) in the machinery industries, while sewing-machine operators making women's clothing averaged well above this amount. Most retail clerks apparently earned less than $1 and women in jobs requiring relatively little skill in some of the chemical industries received about 80 cents, on the average, in July 1946.

Average hourly earnings in nursing were somewhat above those in office jobs into which high-school graduates can go with relatively little specialized training, but were lower than those in office jobs requiring considerable advanced training or experience on the job (such as stenographers who take technical dictation and bookkeepers). In the fall of 1946, when nurses averaged $1 an hour, earnings of women in the office jobs for which data are available varied from roughly 80 cents an hour for clerk-typists to around $1.10–$1.15 for bookkeepers.

Although no group is strictly comparable with nurses, salaries of teachers are of particular interest because of the high proportion of women in both professions and the fact that the average time spent on education by members of the two fields is about the same. (However, the cash expenditure required for teachers' training is generally much above that of nurses.) Salaries of teachers in city school systems were distinctly higher than those of nurses, but inclusion of rural school salaries would probably about equalize the average salary of nurses and of teachers. Assuming full employment, nurses' annual salaries were about $2,100 a year while the average for city school teachers was about $2,500 annually in the 1946–47 school year. If the very large group of teachers in rural schools were included, a comparable figure would, it is estimated, be about $2,100 for the same period.

Earnings of California medical laboratory technicians, who had more education and experience than the average nurse, were apparently above those of California nurses, but in New York State, staff nurses' salaries seemed to be on a level with those of laboratory technicians. Medical laboratory technicians in California received average weekly salaries of about $50 in January 1946. These technicians typically had a bachelor's degree and averaged about 8 years of experience in their work. (Nurses in California earned around $50 a week about 9 months later.) A study of workers in New York State made in July and August 1946 showed average annual earnings of hospital staff nurses to be on a level with those of X-ray technicians, occupational and physical therapists, and laboratory technicians but below those of social workers and of workers in relatively responsible clerical positions.

Those participants in the present study who had left nursing for other fields of employment earned an average of $188 a month, about $12 above nurses' cash earnings.

Hours and other working conditions. Hours and other working conditions in and outside the nursing field at the time of the Bureau's study can be roughly compared as follows:

1. Hours of work were shorter and more regular outside nursing than in most branches of the profession. Women in office work and in most manufacturing plants typically worked about 40 hours a week. There were exceptions, particularly in retail trade, where 48-hour schedules were fairly widespread. Information on hours of teachers was difficult to obtain, particularly because of the time they spend on school work outside regular classroom hours. Inactive nurses who had gone into other jobs averaged about 41 hours weekly in October 1946, compared with a 44-hour average for those who had remained in nursing. Time on call and split shifts, still found to a substantial extent in nursing, were unusual in other fields into which large numbers of women go.

2. Proportionately fewer women in industry worked at night than did nurses and they more frequently received premium pay when they did go on the night shift.

3. In contrast to nurses and teachers, workers in industrial establishments generally received overtime pay at time and a half their regular rate. Teachers fared less well in overtime provisions than nurses, who sometimes got some compensation for overtime.

4. Paid vacations and sick leave were more widespread and liberal for nurses than for workers in industry. Teachers had even longer vacations and fared about as well as nurses in sick leave arrangements. Vacations of industrial workers were most commonly 1 week in length after 1 year's service while 2-week vacations were most frequent for office workers. Longer vacations were unusual for industrial or office workers and they were generally not covered by sick leave plans. The great majority of California medical technicians received vacations (frequently from 10 to 20 days in length) and sick leave.

5. Nurses did not fare as well in provisions for retirement as most other groups for which comparative data were available. City school teachers were generally covered by retirement pension plans; also over two-thirds of the California medical technicians were included in such plans. Most workers in American industry are covered by the retirement and unemployment compensation provisions of the Social Security Act.

Obviously if nursing was to remain an attractive profession for women, some radical changes had to be made. As the following article would indicate, the situation had not been greatly improved in 1962.

27.
Medicine's Forgotten Women

by Barbara Carter

The mounting concern over the nation's health would seem to indicate that at last we are taking the issue seriously. President Kennedy has put medical care for the aged in top place among "legislation that must be passed by Congress this year." The U.S. Public Health Survey has just begun its first intensive examination into the general public's health. And Congress has authorized (once again) more spending for medical research than the administration requested.

But the welfare of nurses, whose role is an essential one in nearly all health services, has not been the subject of much public concern. The consequences of such apathy are beginning to tell, and nurses in several states, including Illinois, Tennessee, and California, have taken the unprecedented step of resigning en masse to protest their employment conditions. Meanwhile, the nursing shortage has risen to twenty per cent, doubling the vacancy rate since 1958, and the percentage of high-school graduates entering the profession has dropped significantly. Some hospitals, such as Fordham and Greenpoint in New York, have been ordered closed for lack of nurses, and some new wings have never been used for the same reason. Yet the public apparently still takes the nurses for granted, and the nurses have thus far been unable to do much about it.

A few figures are in order. Almost two-thirds of the nation's 504,000 active registered nurses are employed in hospitals, and sixty per cent of these are general-duty nurses, the position where the most vacancies are reported. The average salary earned by a nurse at this level in a nongovernmental hospital is $3,900. (The situation is somewhat better all around in government hospitals, but private nonprofit hospitals employ more than two-thirds of all hospital nurses.) The average factory worker earns almost a thousand dollars a year more—$4,730. And the average classroom teacher,

From *The Reporter*. March 1, 1962, 35–37.

whose economic distress have been widely publicized in recent years, earns what suddenly appears to be a generous $5,215 a year. The wage of a New York City bus driver, which was raised to $108 a week after the New Year's Day strike, is appreciably more, especially with overtime pay, than the national average of $103.85 for the top hospital nursing position, that of nursing director.

Money, however, is only part of the picture. The large majority of nurses do not have unemployment insurance, do not get time and a half for overtime, do not get compulsory Social Security coverage, and do not have a voice in determining their own working conditions. Very few of them have been able to engage in the type of collective bargaining that leads to a negotiated contract. If their benefits haven't increased, their burdens have, particularly in the added numbers of auxiliary personnel to supervise.

After the Second World War, while standards of living were generally moving upward in the United States, nurses found themselves at an unusual disadvantage. In 1946, their professional organization, the American Nurses' Association, which was founded in 1896 to foster high standards of nursing practice and education, initiated an "Economic Security Program." Nurses, who are especially sensitive about their status as members of a profession, still find it difficult to engage in what they prefer to call "union-like" activity, and at the beginning of their program they voluntarily gave up the right to strike. At the same time, however, the ANA trained its state association officers to serve as representatives—when asked—to negotiate with employers on salaries, hours, and so forth. By 1947, it had been able to negotiate contracts and engage in collective bargaining in three or four states. But then came the Taft-Hartley Act, which for the first time specifically excluded nonprofit hospitals, or half of the country's hospitals, from the legal obligation to bargain collectively. Since then, the nurses' representatives have been able to negotiate contracts in a total of only seven states.

The Taft-Hartley bill's reference to hospitals, which had been sponsored by the American Hospital Association and Johns Hopkins Hospital, was slipped in from the floor by the late Senator Millard Tydings of Maryland, and adopted with practically no debate.

In prior hearings, the Hospital Association had argued that patients' fees and charitable contributions were not a "proper" subject for collective bargaining, and that citizens should be protected from strikes against nonprofit hospitals. The latter point, as far as nurses are concerned, was irrelevant, since they had already given up the right to strike. The president of Johns Hopkins Hospital had pointed to a somewhat mystical connection between the community and the hospital (". . . in effect simply two parts of the same entity") and concluded that "It would, therefore, seem highly unethical and detrimental to the public welfare for [a] hospital . . . to be compelled to bargain with a stated group or labor union. . . ."

Senator Tydings may not have understood the A.H.A.'s maneuver. When he offered his amendment, he was asked only one question: "What does the amendment do . . . ? Does it prevent hospital employees, particularly nurses, from organizing . . . ?" "I do not think it would," Mr. Tydings replied, and added, "I do not think the amendment will affect them in the slightest way as to salaries. I will say . . . they can still protest, they can still walk out." With this assurance, the Senate promptly adopted his amendment.

Since then, hospital administrators have tended to act as if the exclusion not only frees them from any legal requirement to bargain collectively, which it does, but also as if it forbids them to negotiate with nurses' representatives, which it doesn't.

If the nurses ever succeed in getting the clause out of the labor act (and the AFL-CIO itself is reluctant to bring up the subject of changes just now) and if its removal were to prompt the nine states that have added the provision to their labor laws to do the same, the most the nurses could hope for would be a better chance to state their case. The real issues would still have to be fought out, and here the nurses are very much alone against a highly organized and formidable opponent, the American Hospital Association. Moreover, the nurses are divided among themselves.

Hemmed in both by Taft-Hartley and their own resolve to avoid the more militant forms of unionism, nurses are left with little alternative but to endure or walk out individually, as Senator Tydings casually suggested. Twenty-four of the forty-six nurses at Kewanee, Illinois, Public Hospital did just that last summer. Their story is instructive.

It began in January, 1961, when Kewanee, a nonprofit hospital, raised patients' fees, explaining that the nurses were getting raises. At that time, the beginning salary for a general-duty nurse at Kewanee was $235 a month, $79 below the state average for beginning nurses. In March, after the nurses had pointedly inquired about the heralded raise, the administrator of the hospital offered them a tempting choice: either a salary increase with a fifty per cent cut in the nursing staff, or the same salary with the same number on the staff. The nurses chose the latter.

In April, however, a raise was given, but by that time the nurses, through information supplied by the state branch of the ANA, were more aware of their position relative to the rest of the state. Their average salary, after the raise, came only to $279, while the going rate for nurses in the state was $333. At this point seventy-five per cent of the hospital's nurses decided to make their state association their bargaining agent.

As a first step, they undertook a systematic study of their situation. They discovered that some of the hospital's practices violated state licensing laws, and were in the process of surveying current salaries on the nursing staff when the hospital administration fired the nurse who was gathering this basic information.

The ANA representative and the local chairman thereupon asked the hospital administrator for a meeting, which was refused in line with the Illinois State Hospital Association's policy that "funds allocated for the care of patients will not be subject to bargaining with third parties representing only employee interests. . . ." "The legal precedent for this policy," it was explained, "has been clearly established by the exemption granted hospitals" by the Taft-Hartley Act.

The Kewanee board, however, agreed to meet with the nurses on condition they not bring along an ANA representative.

They met on June 20. On the one side sat the owners of three local businesses, a bank representative, a traffic manager, a personnel manager, and two attorneys; on the other, a few nurses chosen as spokesmen by their group. Before the women could make any presentation of their grievances, they were told that the board would not deal with them as a group but only on an individual basis.

Up against what seemed a blank wall, twenty-four nurses resigned, carefully spacing out their departures. Their decision was not made without a great deal of soul-searching, and the repercussions were nation-wide. Not only was the story covered in the state press, but the hospital's version received full play in the Illinois Hospital Association's newsletter, which in turn was picked up verbatim by the New York Hospital Association and carried in a number of other states' hospital newsletters. It almost sounded like a call to arms.

Despite the formidable opposition massed against them, seventeen of twenty-four nurses working for below-average salaries without night differential or overtime pay in a Southern hospital (which will not be identified here because of possible reprisals against the nurses) decided to ask their state branch of the ANA to assist them as bargaining agent. The administrator's reply to the ANA was brief: "I have no intention of permitting third-party interference in the management of this hospital when no conflict exists in any department. . . ." The administrator lost no time in notifying the state Hospital Association that trouble was brewing. It duly sent a letter to each administrator of all the member hospitals in the state inviting them to meetings to discuss ways to implement their resoluion against collective bargaining. The Kewanee incident was very much on their minds. "In Illinois," the invitation warned, "a similar pattern has developed in one of the hospitals resulting in a number of the nurses resigning from the staff and with full accounts being published in the press on a state-wide basis." Included was a "Statement of Policy to Serve as a Guide to Member Hospitals." Its fifth and final point was: "Each hospital should realize the importance of communicating immediately with the Central Office of [the state] Hospital Association if approached by any group concerned with collective bargaining. The Association will serve as a clearing house and will mobilize such help as may be available from member hospitals informed of developments within the state and maintain liaison with the American Hospital Association."

Earlier, the administrator had written a fatherly letter to the hospital nurse who was chairman of the local unit. "It was," he confessed, ". . . a great disappointment to me to receive a letter from the State Nurses' Association recently in which they state you had instructed them to represent seventeen nurses . . . The [state] Hospital Association and I, as Administrator of this hospital, consider it unnecessary, unethical and ill-advisable to enter into third-party dealings . . . If I might digress for a moment, let me warn you of the communistic influence in this country which is usually spread by parasitic groups that make their living creating dissatisfaction when it does not exist, and appealing to the *greed* of individuals who may act without thinking of its effect on his fellow man. The cycles in history show that benefits gained are paid for by giving greater contributions to these parasitic groups which will lead you through socialism and communism, on to slavery. It has been estimated that if all Graduate Nurses lower themselves to this status, the dues they would pay into the 'slush' fund would be over 24 *million dollars* each year to spend on creating additional discontent."

Having delivered himself of this beguiling intepretation of the history of collective bargaining, the administrator returned to the point of his letter. "How can hospitals respect your ability, sincerity, and loyalty," he asked the nurse, "if your work is guided solely by selfish interests? In conclusion, I wish to advise that if you go through with this ill-advised act, you have lost your professional status and will receive no other consideration than non-professional employees. I urge you to carefully weigh your action in respect to your profession, your hospital, and the people of this city."

In the end, the nurses' professional organization was kept out, though the nurses on their own were able to get some improvement of their position.

And so it goes. In Idaho, four hospital nurses were fired for disloyalty and "gross insubordination" as they attempted to improve their conditions. In Iowa, a Dubuque industrial hospital fired its head nurse and forced two others to resign when they sought assistance from the Iowa Nurses' Association. In Tennessee, the staff nurses of a Nashville hospital, who were getting about $25 a month less than other nurses in the Nashville area but whose protests were of no avail, finally gave two weeks' notice, but got their raise on the date their resignations were to become effective.

Some 280 nurses in eight nonprofit hospitals in Orange County, California, joined the ANA in order to improve their economic condition, to establish better nursing practices, and to persuade the hospitals to enter into collective bargaining with them. The hospitals first offered a $30-a-month increase over the $72.50 weekly starting salary, then brought such pressure to bear that nine nurses were forced to resign and one was fired. Nevertheless, the campaign has had some success: a few hospitals have provided regular salary increases, payment for overtime, and unemployment benefits.

And finally this January, again in Illinois (only 165 miles from Kewanee), all the nurses except the director in a Jerseyville hospital announced their resignations. The issues here were not so much salary as nursing standards, and an unusual feature was the medical staff's support of the nurses. The doctors, in fact, had sent a resolution to the board, noting that routine care of the patients had deteriorated alarmingly and asked that the board fire the administrator. By early February, the administrator had resigned and a settlement of sorts had been reached, but the nurses' state bargaining representative was excluded from the arrangement.

One decisive ANA success should be mentioned here—one that the seemingly more sophisticated members of the labor movement might well envy. The Nurses' Association has found a more effective means of bringing in Southern Negro members than many more experienced labor leaders can boast. They took them directly into their national association when the local Southern organizations demurred, and today all their state branches accept Negroes as members.

In spite of the increasing number of courageous but isolated acts of protest by the nurses, their national organization wonders, "How far can we push them when we have no way to protect them?" Moreover, by no means all nurses are behind their professional organization. Not only do their environment and the pressures they face militate against active outspoken support, but their national organization has suddenly dropped its cloistered role as handmaiden to the American Medical Association and come out independently for medical care for the aged under Social Security, Federal aid to higher education, and a stepped-up "Economic Security Program."

"Now we're on everybody's hate list," was the remark of one ANA member, ruefully acknowledging that ANA membership has dropped suddenly as a result. In 1958, when it first took its stand on Federal care for the aged, its membership totaled 190,463. Today it stands at 170,000.

The ANA's independence on these matters has jolted the A.M.A. is much as the positions themselves. In 1959, one considerate member of the

Florida Medical Association supplied a formal resolution for the state nurses' group to use in reversing their stand on Federal care for the aged. Though they turned it down flat, the same tactic has been tried in other states. Last spring it was reported in *Medical World News* that a special meeting of A.M.A. officials and state leaders had decided "to work on the grass roots level to get local nursing groups to repudiate the ANA endorsement of the Social Security approach to aged care coverage."

"Why aren't nurses our allies any more?" Dr. Alfred P. Ingegno asks in the November 6, 1961, issue of *Medical Economics,* which is described as a "business magazine for doctors." He pointed to the charge that ". . . in some areas doctors have been putting pressure on nurses to bend them to medicine's point of view" and recommended that "we should support the ANA's effort to improve the salaries and working conditions of nurses in hospitals. . . . By aligning ourselves with the nursing profession as it strives for adequate recognition, doctors will be serving an urgent national need for more nurses. . . . It's obvious that the most natural way to stimulate interest in nursing careers is by keeping the nursing profession satisfied, both professionally and economically. It's a better way than scholarships, subsidies, government programs, and pep talks. All these get endless discussion, while everyone—doctors included—turns his back on the hard economic facts of nursing life."

The doctor's remarks touch on a difficult point. Though having the same needs as other employed persons, the nurses are inhibited to a large degree by their concern for their patients and by their determination to maintain their status as professionals. Yet in spite of the stiff professional opposition against them, they have come out strongly for the Kennedy administration's stand on Federal care for the aged and Federal aid to higher education.

For its part, Washington's only recent actions on this serious matter have been a drive to recruit nurses among Indians to be trained in New Mexico and a four-cent stamp honoring the nursing profession.

It is evident from a 1963 survey of the Bureau of Labor Statistics (which permits comparisons with the 1946 report) that organized nursing still has a long way to go before it will be able to significantly better the economic conditions of nurses.

28.
The Continuing Economic Difficulties of Nurses

by Evelyn B. Moses

The economic status of the registered nurse in today's hospital and particularly that of the general duty nurse is of paramount importance in the economic level of nursing in general, because an overwhelming number of nurses are involved.

Despite the number of other areas in which nurses practice today, hospitals and related institutions continue to employ an ever-increasing proportion—over two thirds—of the professional nurses working in this country. Furthermore, almost two fifths of all working nurses are general duty nurses in hospitals.

That the economic base is low is shown in results of a survey announced a few months ago by the Bureau of Labor Statistics of the U.S. Department of Labor. This survey of employment conditions of employees in nonfederal short-term hospitals in metropolitan areas in the country, undertaken in mid-1963, was limited to hospitals of 100 or more employees. Therefore, it excluded small hospitals in metropolitan areas as well as all hospitals, both large and small, in nonmetropolitan areas. It also excluded all psychiatric and tuberculosis hospitals as well as sanitoriums and other long-term hospitals and institutions. A total of 1,624 hospitals employing 970,140 workers, including about 138,000 full-time professional registered nurses, came within the scope of the survey. About four fifths of the employees were in nongovernment hospitals and one fifth in the state and local government hospitals.

Salary Ranges

The average salaries of professional registered nurses in the hospitals of the type studied ranged from $86.50 per week for general duty nurses to $152.00 for directors of nursing. Head nurses averaged $98.50; supervisors, $110.50; and instructors, $105.00.

Nurses as a group fared best in the West where salaries were the highest. The lowest salaries were found in the South and salary levels in the north central area, in most instances, were slightly higher than those in the northeastern area. Salary levels also were generally higher in state and local government hospitals, larger metropolitan areas, and in larger hospitals. In the last instance, there were greater differences among the higher level nursing

From "Nursing's Economic Plight". Reprinted, with permission, from *The American Journal of Nursing, 65,* January 1965, 68–71.

AVERAGE WEEKLY EARNINGS IN NONFEDERAL SHORT-TERM HOSPITALS IN METROPOLITAN AREAS, MIDYEAR 1963*					
Type of Position	United States	Northeast	South	North Central	West
Director of nursing	$152.00	$160.50	$137.50	$148.00	$159.00
Supervisor of nurses	110.50	113.00	98.50	113.50	120.50
Nursing instructors	105.00	107.00	96.50	107.00	111.50
Head nurse	98.50	101.50	86.00	100.50	107.50
General duty nurse	86.50	85.50	77.00	88.50	93.50

* The survey covered nonfederal government and nongovernmental short-term hospitals with 100 or more employees located in the nation's Standard Metropolitan Statistical Areas as defined by the U.S. Bureau of the Budget in 1961. Tuberculosis and psychiatric hospitals were excluded from the survey.

positions, particularly that of the director of nursing, than among the lower level nursing positions. For example, in areas of one million or more population the average salary of a general duty nurse in a nongovernment hospital with under 500 employees was $89.00 and in a hospital with 500 or more employees, it was $89.50. The comparable averages for directors of nursing were $143.00 and $173.00.

A frequent question in any discussion of nursing salaries is what differentials exist between the various levels of nursing positions. The average salary of head nurses in the United States was 14 percent higher than that of general duty nurses. Instructors averaged 21 percent more than general duty nurses; supervisors averaged 28 percent more, and directors of nursing 76 percent more.

However, these differentials are not uniform throughout the country nor from hospital to hospital. In nongovernment hospitals head nurses averaged 13 percent more than general duty nurses; directors of nursing, 75 percent more. In state and local government hospitals, head nurses averaged 16 percent more and directors of nursing 80 percent more. The widest differentials among professional nursing positions generally were found in the northeastern sector of the country. As noted before, differentials were also greater in the larger hospitals than in the smaller ones. No matter how finely hospitals are classified, variations in differentials between positions still exist. No mathematical formula is applied in all instances. Obviously, many other factors are involved.

Comparisons in the Hospital

In the Bureau of Labor Statistics study, which covered other professional and technical occupations as well as nonprofessional occupations, the average salary of general duty nurses was next to the lowest of all the professional and technical occupations studied. The exception was that of x-ray technicians. X-ray technicians averaged $82.50 a week, while, as previously indicated, the general duty nurse averaged $86.50. Head nurses also averaged less than the other groups with two exceptions, the x-ray technician, of course, and the medical technologist. Head nurses also averaged less than the stationary engineers, maintenance electricians, and chief housekeepers. While the supervisors averaged more than such groups as the medical record librarians, the physical therapists, and the dietitians, they averaged less than chief x-ray technicians and the medical social workers. Next to the director of nursing, the medical social worker was the highest paid of the professional positions studied.

Licensed practical nurses averaged $64.50 a week, 74 percent of the average salary of the general duty nurse, and nursing aides averaged $53.50, which was 62 percent of the average salary of the general duty nurse in this report.

As was true for the levels within professional nursing, varying differentials were also found in comparing professional nursing and other hospital occupations. For example, while general duty nurses in the country as a whole averaged 34 percent more than the licensed practical nurses, they averaged only 26 percent more in the northeastern sector and 43 percent more in the southern area. General duty nurses in the country averaged 62 percent more than nursing aides, but in the northeastern area they averaged 46 percent more and in the southern area 90 percent more.

Of interest in relation to the factors involved in establishing salary levels and the differences between levels for the various occupations, is a comparison of 1963 and 1960 pay levels in four positions in nongovernmental hospitals in 15 metropolitan areas included in the Bureau of Labor Statistics report.* This shows that the highest proportionate increase—19 percent—in the general duty nurse's average salary occurred in New York City. The maids in New York City experienced a 30 percent increase; the nursing aides, a 26 percent increase; and the practical nurses, a 20 percent increase. In Portland, Oregon, where there was only a 9 percent increase in the average salary of general duty nurses, there was an even lower proportionate in-

* The areas covered are: Atlanta, Baltimore, Boston, Buffalo, Chicago, Cincinnati, Cleveland, Dallas, Los Angeles-Long Beach, Memphis, Minneapolis-St. Paul, New York City, Philadelphia, Portland (Oregon), San Francisco-Oakland.

crease—7 percent—in the average salary of the nursing aides. Obviously, differentials between occupational groups shift since the rate of salary adjustment which one group may experience from time to time is not necessarily the same as another's.

Comparisons Outside Hospitals

Using the figures from this survey, one can readily see that nursing salaries today are far below those of other professional occupations. Nurses are frequently compared to teachers in the public school system because teaching is to a large extent a female occupation and the one which has been traditionally considered nursing's "rival" as a career to which women who go on to post high school education will be attracted. The National Education Association estimates the average salary of classroom teachers in 1963-1964 to be $5,963. This is $217 above the average salary of the nurse supervisor in the BLS study, and $1,465 above the average salary of the general duty nurse. However, despite gains that teachers have made in recent years, teaching, like nursing, is still among the lower paid professional groups. Even greater discrepancies are found when comparisons are made between nursing and other professions.

In a study which the Bureau of Labor Statistics made in private industry in early 1963, the average salary of an accountant in a beginning position with minimum educational requirements of a baccalaureate degree was shown as $6,156. This is $1,658 above the average salary of the general duty nurse. The average salary of engineers in this level of position was $7,056, $2,558 above the average salary of the general duty nurse and only $848 below the average salary of the director of nursing. This same study showed an average salary of $8,952 for a personnel director in charge of a relatively small work force, $1,048 above the average salary of the director of nursing.

A characteristic job of women, one that does not necessarily require post high school education, is that of secretary. A Bureau of Labor Statistics survey in metropolitan areas showed an average weekly salary of $96.50 for secretaries in February 1963. This was $10.00 higher than the average salary of general duty nurses in the BLS survey of metropolitan area hospitals. In an area such as Atlanta, the average weekly salary of secretaries was almost $20.00 higher than that of general duty nurses.

Beyond Salaries

Salaries alone are not enough to determine the working conditions of a group and any evaluation should also take into account fringe benefits and other conditions. In all but one of these areas—vacations—nurses on the whole do not fare as well as other employees.

One of the basic provisions of the employment standards for general duty nurses as established in most of the state nurses' associations is that there be an established salary range with progression from the minimum to the maximum salary to be determined by length of service. The Bureau of Labor Statistics study shows that 95 percent of the general duty nurses in nongovernment hospitals and 99 percent in state and local government hospitals were employed under a formal salary system. However, only 48 percent of the nongovernment nurses under these systems received length-of-service increments while 59 percent of the government nurses were employed under such increment plans. Further examination of the salary schedule provisions for general duty nurses shows a wide variation in established minimum salaries among hospitals in the country with even more variation among government than nongovernment hospitals. Although there was little difference in the number of steps in the ranges—half of the general duty nurses in government hospitals and 48 percent of the general duty nurses in nongovernment hospitals were under plans with at least six steps—government hospitals tended to have wider salary ranges than nongovernment.

For the most part, according to the survey, professional nurses worked 40 hours a week. About 6 percent of the nurses in nongovernment hospitals and 3 percent in government hospitals were scheduled to work less than 40 hours a week. Among the other professional or technical workers in the hospitals, about 12 percent in nongovernment hospitals and 21 percent in government hospitals were scheduled to work less than 40 hours a week. Data on office workers in private industry in metropolitan areas for 1962-1963 show that 36 percent of these workers had scheduled work weeks of less than 40 hours.

Holidays

Nurses usually received at least five paid holidays a year. In nongovernment hospitals about 53 percent of the nurses received at least seven paid holidays. Once again the South, where holiday provisions were the least liberal, trailed behind other regions of the country. Holiday provisions were most liberal in the northeastern area. Also once again, conditions were best in government hospitals which provided more paid holidays than were provided in nongovernment hospitals.

Office workers in the nation's metropolitan areas tended to have more paid holidays than nurses in hospitals, with 77 percent receiving at least seven paid holidays a year.

Among office workers, as in the case of nurses, holiday provisions were better than the national picture in the Northeast and lowest in the South.

However, 59 percent of the office workers in the Northeast received at least nine holidays a year while in nongovernment hospitals in the Northeast, only 33 percent of the nurses received at least nine paid holidays a year. In the South, about 38 percent of the nurses had less than six holidays a year. Only 3 percent of the office workers had less than six holidays a year.

Vacations

Most nurses received at least two weeks' vacation with pay after one year of service. About 22 percent of the nurses in nongovernment hospitals and 24 percent in government hospitals received at least three weeks' vacation with pay after one year. After five years of service, 66 percent of the nongovernment hospital nurses and 64 percent of the government hospital nurses received at least three weeks' vacation with pay. Over 85 percent of the nurses received at least three weeks' vacation with pay after 10 years of service with over a third receiving four weeks after 10 years. Examination of data available on office workers shows that nurses tend to have better vacation provisions. No data were available on vacations for professional employees in industry.

Health Insurance

The areas of health insurance and retirement benefits for which the employer provides part or all of the coverage are other fringe benefits in which nurses generally do not fare as well as office workers in private industry. Life insurance was available to 96 percent of the office workers. This type of insurance was available to only 44 percent of the nongovernment hospital nurses and 47 percent of the state and local government hospital nurses. Although nurses were covered by sick-leave plans while only 67 percent of office workers had such coverage, much larger proportions of office workers were covered by accidental death and dismemberment insurance and sickness and accident insurance. Hospitalization insurance was available to 44 percent of the nongovernment nurses and 56 percent of the government nurses. When you add to these proportions those who received free or reduced cost care in the hospital the proportions become 87 percent and 77 percent. Eighty-six percent of the office workers in private industry in metropolitan areas were covered by hospitalization insurance. Eighty-five percent of the office workers had surgical insurance plans available to them and 69 percent had medical insurance available. The combination of surgical insurance and/or care provided outside of insurance was available to only 49 percent of nongovernment hospital nurses and only 65 percent of government hospital nurses. Medical benefits were also available to lesser proportions of hospital nurses than they were to office workers.

Retirement Benefits

Ninety-three percent of the nongovernment hospital nurses in the
BLS study and 94 percent of the state and local government hospital nurses
were covered by social security and/or some other retirement pension plan.
Social security coverage was reported for 89 percent of the nongovernment
hospital nurses and 62 percent of the government hospital nurses. Among
hospital nurses, 42 percent of the nongovernment nurses and 51 percent of
the government nurses were covered by social security and another retirement
plan. In contrast, 78 percent of the office workers covered by the BLS study
in metropolitan areas in 1962-1963 were covered by retirement pension
plans other than social security. These employers are required to cover workers
by social security. It is not mandatory within the social security act for
nonprofit and government hospital employers to cover their employees.

HEALTH, INSURANCE AND RETIREMENT PLANS
(Percent of workers)

Type of Plan	U.S. Hospital Nurses (mid-1963)		U.S. Office Workers (1962-1963)
	Nongov't.	Gov't.	
Life insurance	44	47	96
Accidental death and dismemberment insurance	25	25	56
Sickness and accident insurance	12	4	40
Sick leave (full or partial)	99	99	67
Hospitalization insurance[a]	44	56	86
Surgical insurance[b]	33	52	85
Medical insurance[c]	27	49	69
Catastrophe insurance (major medical)	8	34	61
Social security and other retirement	42	51	78

[a] A total of 87 percent of the nongovernment hospital nurses and 77 of the government hospital nurses received some hospitalization benefits either through care outside of insurance or insurance or both.

[b] A total of 49 percent of the nongovernment hospital nurses and 65 percent of the government hospital nurses received some surgical benefits either through care outside of insurance or insurance or both.

[c] A total of 51 percent of the nongovernment hospital nurses and 62 percent of the government hospital nurses received some medical benefits either through care outside of insurance or insurance or both.

This brief review of the data contained in the studies made by the Bureau of Labor Statistics shows that employment conditions for professional nurses do not measure up to those of other occupational groups. Obviously, in salaries, fringe benefits, and other conditions of employment, nursing today cannot compete with many occupations and professions which are now open to women aside from those which have been traditionally female. This is particularly detrimental to nursing today when funds are available to many more people for post high school education. Certainly, this affects recruitment into the profession adversely and bodes ill for efforts to maintain, much less to increase, the level of nurse supply for the years ahead.

It also almost negates efforts being made to attract back into active practice those nurses who are presently inactive. A large proportion of the nurses in this group are married and in the younger age brackets and cite home and family responsibilities as major reasons for not working. Unquestionably, $4,500 a year cannot cover the cost of arrangements necessary to take care of home and family responsibilities as well as provide additional income for the families of these nurses. Under such conditions, returning to work can hardly be considered financially attractive to inactive nurses.

> Nursing, like many other professional groups, has been plagued with the problem of securing economic status to match its services. Individual nurses quite obviously cannot do it by themselves, but group action might. Other professional groups have actively organized to protect their economic interests, and nurses might well imitate some of their actions.

29.
Economic Activity Among Various Professional Groups

by Joel Seidman

The trend today for professional groups to actively protect their economic interests seems to me unmistakable. There is space here only to review, briefly, the experience of some groups of salaried professionals in this. In the case of teachers, for example, the chief problem has been a low level of

From "The Trend Among Professional Groups Today." Reprinted, with permission, from *The American Journal of Nursing*, LXV January 1965, 72–75.

salaries. The research department of the National Education Association reports that male teachers in elementary and high schools averaged only $5,500 in 1961, that almost half worked at two jobs, and that 60 percent took summer employment. Another problem of teachers is that, for the most part, they are public employees, and in some states the organization of public employees, or negotiation with them, is prohibited by law. Strikes of public employees are generally prohibited by both federal and state law. In addition, there are financial complications such as the raising of funds by taxation, the allocation of revenue to school expense by authority other than the head of the school system, and the governing of expenditures by a budget that teachers cannot readily influence.

In the teaching field there are two leading organizations, the National Education Association founded in 1857, and the American Federation of Teachers formed in 1916. The NEA, a professional society that includes both administrators and teachers, is, for this reason, hardly suited for collective bargaining. It raises a question as to the freedom of teachers to oppose administrators within the organization and it may also involve administrators in conflict-of-interest situations. The AFT, formed frankly to function as a labor organization, promptly affiliated with the American Federation of Labor, and now is an affiliate of the merged AFL-CIO.

Traditionally the NEA has opposed collective bargaining for teachers, though it has favored representations by teachers on salaries and other issues of interest to them. As a result of the wartime and postwar inflation, however, the NEA has encouraged its local affiliates to represent teachers in bargaining. In 1962 the NEA, announcing its support of "professional negotiation" by teachers while continuing to oppose collective bargaining, called for participation by teachers with boards of education in the determination of policies of mutual concern. Though continuing to oppose the strike, the NEA favors utilization of "professional sanctions," under which members in the locality are advised to seek employment elsewhere, while members employed elsewhere are warned that acceptance of employment in that school district is unethical behavior that could result in expulsion from the NEA. In Utah in 1963, following this policy, the state NEA affiliate threatened that teachers would not return to their posts unless state spending for public schools was increased.

In the last several years, as the demand of teachers in some metropolitan areas for bargaining recognition has become more insistent, the NEA has further modified its attitude. In New York City, for example, the AFT local in November 1960, conducted a one-day strike to support its demand for a collective bargaining election. When the election was held the teachers voted, despite NEA opposition, for collective bargaining. In December

1961, the AFT local was chosen over the NEA unit as the collective bargaining agency for the 42,000 teachers. In the bargaining that followed, the AFT local won substantial salary increases amounting to $995 for most teachers, besides obtaining relief for teachers from clerical and other non-professional chores, the appointment of special guidance and reading teachers for problem children, and the establishment of a grievance procedure ending in arbitration. In September 1963, the AFT local in New York called off a scheduled strike as it won further salary gains and a limit in the size of classes.

New York City's is not the only such case. In Detroit, after voting overwhelmingly for exclusive representation by the majority union, the teachers, in May 1964, selected the AFT local over the NEA affiliate as bargaining agency. In Milwaukee, on the other hand, the NEA unit won exclusive bargaining rights, defeating the AFT. Currently, AFT locals are striving for bargaining recognition in Los Angeles, District of Columbia, Chicago, and other centers, while in Wisconsin towns NEA and AFT affiliates are opposing each other for bargaining rights under a new state law. In other areas, where there are no formal recognition or collective bargaining negotiations, NEA or AFT units exert varying degrees of influence on school boards and administrators with regard to salary scales and other issues.

Another interesting group of professionals is composed of engineers and scientists. Though unions of engineers have existed as far back as 1919, the first real growth occurred after World War II, when engineers were employed in establishments in large numbers, out of direct contact with top management. This trend, if anything, continues to accelerate. One of the leading grievances of engineers in the postwar period was a telescoping of salaries— a tendency to raise the pay of beginning engineers in a tight labor market without comparable increases going to experienced engineers.

Professional engineering societies have traditionally opposed unionization of engineers and collective bargaining as unprofessional. However, significant change occurred in 1943-1944 when the American Society of Civil Engineers, alarmed by NLRB rules putting engineers in bargaining units dominated by blue collar workers, promoted the formation of employee committees for collective bargaining. In 1952 an independent union, the Engineers and Scientists of America, was formed by 9 local unions of engineers with 14,000 members and representation rights for 25,000. However, this organization split over the admission of technicians and it has since dissolved, though some of its constituent units still exist.

In 1960 the National Science Foundation estimated that, while 40,000 of the 750,000 engineers in the United States were represented by unions, only 20,000 of these were dues-paying members, and fewer than 7,500 belonged to affiliates of the AFL-CIO. Market conditions have been favorable to engineers in recent years, with a resulting rise in salaries. The professional engineering societies continue to campaign against unionism, arguing that it is incompatible with professionalism, and urging instead that nonbargaining "sounding boards" be established to improve communication between engineers and management.

In their collective bargaining objectives unions of engineers tend to differ markedly from blue collar groups. While many of the objectives are similar, unions of engineers place far more emphasis on individual merit, favoring this rather than seniority as a basis for promotion, and generally seeking pay increases, at least in part, on a merit basis. Engineering unions show great interest in measures to improve the professional competence of their members, such as payment for time off to attend professional society meetings, partial refund by management of tuition fees for professional courses, and payment by management of dues in professional societies. Unions of engineers generally do not seek the union shop, a prime objective of most blue collar unions.

Other professional groups have organized for collective bargaining activities. One of these, the Actors Equity Association, was formed in 1919 when it conducted a successful 30-day strike for recognition. Actors suffered from a number of grievances at that time, including unpaid rehearsals lasting weeks or even months, the need to pay for their own costumes, the danger of being stranded when touring shows failed, and the lack of arbitration machinery. Actors in films are organized into the Screen Actors Guild, which was formed in 1933 to protest a sharp pay cut. Long-standing complaints of screen actors at that time included insufficient rest between calls, and the lack of overtime pay or of premium pay for Saturdays, Sundays, holidays, and night work.

The musicians' union was already powerful when the Actors Equity was launched in 1919. A major problem of the musicians for many years has been the availability of canned music, reducing the demand for live performers. The musicians have sought to meet this problem by a royalty on records, the proceeds being used to support free concerts. Another problem confronting many serious musicians who are members of symphony orchestras is that they are employed by nonprofit organizations operating at a deficit. In some cases in recent years union pressure has concentrated on lengthening the playing season, with the result that the 52-week year, including paid vacations was finally achieved in the 1964 contracts with such leading musical organizations as the New York Philharmonic, the Philadelphia Orchestra, and the Cleveland Orchestra. Musicians, unlike most other groups of unionists, face a delicate problem of achieving reasonable job security while safeguarding the artistic standards of the organization. They also are confronted with an unusual internal union problem, arising from the presence of large numbers of part-time musicians, vastly outnumbering—and hence readily able to outvote—the minority of union members who are dependent on music for their livelihood.

A highly unusual union group is composed of airline pilots, whose leading members now earn over $30,000 yearly. The chief function of the Air Line Pilots' Association, formed in 1930, has been to increase the earnings of its members. Hours present no problem, since maximum flying hours have long been set at 85 monthly by government decision. The association also engages in research and consultative work on safety, new equipment, airport facilities, air traffic control, and the like—the professional side of its activities.

The union of reporters, the American Newspaper Guild, also deserves mention. It was formed in 1933, as a response to a wave of newspaper mergers that reduced employment. This difficulty was compounded by the fact that salaries for reporters were lower than the pay scales of unionized newspaper employees doing mechanical work such as typesetting.

Collective bargaining has even made its appearance among physicians, whose standing as professionals is surely unimpeachable. Yet salaried employment of physicians, where it occurs, brings problems comparable to those faced by salaried employees with other types of skills. Problems arose with the Department of Health in New York City, which employs 1,000 public health physicians and dentists, who became concerned over issues such as salary increases, tenure, and higher pensions. In 1961, as a result, they formed the Doctors Association of the New York City Department of Health, the first collective bargaining association of physicians in the United States.

Among the other problems confronting some groups of professional workers is that their work is peculiarly related to public health, making the tactic of withdrawal of service, so effective with blue collar unionists, difficult or impossible to employ. Professionals may work for nonprofit private agencies, many of which suffer chronic deficits and all of which find it difficult or perhaps impossible to pass on increased costs in the manner of private business concerns. Still other professionals are exempt from both federal and state labor legislation, or they are employed by public agencies, where the right to strike does not exist and where salaries may be determined by legislation, restricting the scope of collective bargaining where such activity is permitted.

Under some circumstances, individual action suffices to solve the problems confronting professionals. Individual action is unlikely to be effective, however, where professionals are salaried employees, where they are employed in large numbers in big organizations, and where market factors are not favorable. And, these conditions are true of most professional employees today. It follows that, where these conditions exist, some form of group action must be undertaken if the problems confronting professional workers are to be solved.

Any of the solutions mentioned earlier can be defended, if it is competent to solve the economic problems confronting the group and if it appeals most strongly to the people concerned. One should recognize, however, that attitudes often change over time, and that an organizational form that appears unpopular today may be commonplace tomorrow.

My own view is that professional workers need to maximize their power in collective bargaining and their influence over legislation. Management and management-oriented groups are likely to be hostile to group economic action in any event, as the organized labor movement will be sympathetic; so that little will be lost, except perhaps in self-image, by an alliance with the labor movement, whereas the gain in influence, particularly for legislative purposes, might be substantial. Yet such a move would offer most promise of success, given the present attitudes of professional workers, if they had their own organizations and could determine their own objectives and tactics. It goes without saying, in addition, that the particular professional group involved would have to be ready to take this step.

There is a close relationship between professionalism and the solution of economic problems, in that higher salaries, improved working conditions, and greater job security make the field more attractive, and bring and hold better people. The solution of the economic problems confronting a group of professionals permits them to concentrate on their work and do a better professional job. In addition, unions of professionals use collective bargaining, in part, as a way of advancing professional goals. Thus teachers have been able to reduce classroom size, obtain relief from clerical and other nonprofessional duties, and provide special help for problem children. Engineers, similarly, have won company financial support for advanced training and for attendance at meetings of professional societies.

I see nothing wrong with group effort to promote self-interest by helping to solve group economic problems. Professionals who follow this path will solve their problems faster, thus making their profession more attractive, whereas those who fail to utilize group effort are likely to fall behind in an economic sense; this would constitute no contribution, either to the workers in the field or to the public interest.

In recent years an awareness of the economic problems of the profession has grown. First steps were taken in 1946 when the American Nurses Association initiated an economic security program designed to enable state and local nurses associations to bargain for their members. In papers 30 and 31, two nurse writers tell of some of the difficulties encountered by nurses in their efforts to improve their economic position by collective action.

30.
SNA Experiences with Collective Bargaining

by Anne Zimmerman

Nurses Themselves Resist Any Collective Bargaining

I don't think I need to tell you about this attitude—the attitude that it's unprofessional to talk about salaries and conditions of employment. You know what comes up when you sit as a representative of nurses and talk about the rightness of collective action. You know, too, that there are many statements explaining that it is less dignified for the nurse to work under some of the conditions she accepts, than it is for her to do something about it. You know there are all kinds of statements to support this position—from religious-affiliated groups, professional groups, scholars who write on the subject. But deep down underneath, the nurse's attitude that this might bring disfavor from her colleagues, her supervisor, her employer, or the community, is the most difficult thing I think we have to overcome.

In addition to the attitude that this is "something nurses don't do," we also have resistance from nurses in top management positions. Because of the jobs they hold, they are logically representatives of management. Until we—as a profession—can assist them to be more secure in their management positions and to accept the rightness of democratic action on the part of those over whom they have some authority, I don't think we are ever going to overcome their opposition.

Another reason for resistance within our own organization is that nurses are afraid, and rightfully so, unfortunately. They are afraid they'll be isolated by contemporaries who don't approve; afraid of disapproval by their im-

From *Proceedings,* American Nurses' Association Economic Security Conference, New York: ANA, 1961, pp. 27–31.

mediate supervisors; afraid of losing their jobs. Even after a group gets started, if their leader is dismissed or reprimanded in some way, the nurses become uneasy and afraid for their jobs. They may be working in the only hospital in the community and in sticking together to ask for their leader's reinstatement, they may be risking their own jobs. It's not an easy decision to make.

Some nurses resist because they just don't know what their rights and privileges are under the contract. Now we do have nurses who are under civil service systems and nurses under group contract or individual contracts; but how little they know about the protection they really have!

I think it's rather amazing how little nurses know of their rights and privileges as employees. They understand the role in which they function—that of an expert in the field of nursing care and a member of the profession; but they really do not understand their second role—that of an employee of an agency or institution. We need to overcome this lack of understanding not only because lack of information contributes to a lack of courage but also because uniformed courage is really worse than none at all.

Another of our internal problems is that we function in a nonprofit atmosphere. You've heard nurses say: "There are no profits over which to bargain." "The hospital's running in the red." "They are doing this all for charity." "If we ask for an increase in salary, and this means an increase in the hospital's rates, the community will not support this." These nurses are assuming the responsibility of management. They are not thinking of whether or not they need an increase, but of how management is going to pay for it. I'm always so interested in how anxious they are to help the manager solve *his* problem.

You also know that we suffer from a lack of legislative protection; when it comes down to whether or not the hospital has to meet with its employees, there are only a few labor laws in the country that require this. But I also know of protective laws that *do* cover nurses, and that are rejected by them. In the State of Illinois, we have what is known as a "six-day law." It is about the only law that does *not* exempt either hospital workers or nurses, and it really means that *everybody* must have a day of rest after six consecutive days of work. A number of nurses resent that law and wish they weren't under it. They want to work ten days in a row so they can have four consecutive days off. When we announced that this was a violation of the law—the one law that nurses have that protects them, we don't get any protest from the employer, but we did get resistance from nurses. These are some of the things within the profession that we have to cope with.

Employer Resistance to Collective Bargaining

The last and perhaps the most effective area of resistance is the organized, effective opposition of the employers of nurses. This is the one area that needs our concerted attention. The pronouncement of the American Hospital Association on collective bargaining is probably one of the most frequently promulgated statements in this country. The AHA says, quite truthfully, that they don't have jurisdiction over individual hospital members, that they can't speak effectively for them in a way that will be binding. Nonetheless, state hospital associations all over the country have picked up the statement on collective bargaining and have been effective in having it implemented in their member hospitals. And I'm telling you, that unless we have a tool that *is* binding, it is not effective. The hospital association makes tremendous resources available to the individual hospitals that are resisting recognition. Indeed, it was unity within the hospital associations that defeated the efforts of three different unions to unionize the nonprofessional employees in Chicago last year.

There are other ways in which the hospital association is effective. For one, the journals of the hospital association have carried articles (usually by a past president of the American Hospital Association) reminding members that one of the most effective ways to render an organization ineffective is to diminish its financial resources. We can't lose sight of this factor—not when we see decreasing membership in many of the state nurses associations and the American Nurses' Association. When we lose members, we lose the resources that are absolutely necessary for the effective handling of an economic security program. In some areas, nurses are being actively encouraged to join other organizations, touted as substitutes for membership in their professional organization, and to salve their professional conscience in so doing.

Resistance in Retreat

Now, let me talk briefly about overcoming resistance. It is being done. It is our biggest job, and we ought not to leave discouraged, or without hope. Those of you who read the literature regularly must certainly be impressed with the greater acceptance of collective action for employees of nonprofit institutions and the increasing recognition that here is a serious problem that must be solved one way or another. You must be impressed at the community support that can be rallied around an individual who has been a victim of these problems. There is much more support than there was a decade ago when some of us first started working on an economic security program.

There is another thing coming to pass and that is that a number of religious organizations now have positive and forthright statements on the right of the employee to organize and to have a voice in the determination of employment conditions. You can rightfully say to me that many of these are on paper only and meant to stay there; but more and more, the people involved are examining these documents rather carefully, and giving serious attention to the fact that they have a responsibility not only for the patients in their institutions but for the people who care for patients as well. This is going to be a slow process, but it is on the move.

Something else is coming about. I had an opportunity to speak with the Chicago Hospital Council about this program, and I heard the attitudes expressed by a younger, more enlightened, better educated group of hospital administrators. It occurred to me that recognition of the democratic principles of collective action as a force for good within the institution will be given more readily by some of these up-and-coming young men in hospitals, than by some of our own members. As a force from outside, it will have an influence on us as we strive to eliminate the resistance from within our own organization. The ongoing educational programs of the American Nurses' Association, the SNA's (State Nurses' Associations), district associations, sections, show our responsibility in this area.

The universities are becoming more and more interested in our economic security program. People at the universities are becoming more and more knowledgeable in this field and, as the information gets down into our own organization and eventually into the place where it really belongs—in the school of nursing—this will also be a potent force for good and for overcoming resistance from within our profession. The development of leadership among nurses is going to help.

At first, the words "collective bargaining" were unacceptable; now they are part of the ANA platform. This is action that points the real direction for this program.

I honestly think that as we move away from the image of Florence Nightingale, living on the oil in her lamp, toward the image of the nurse as a responsible, educated member of the community, entitled to a voice in her employment conditions, and a living wage, that we will change *resistance* to *insistence*.

31.
The Situation in Nursing

by Dorothy Kelly

In the Book of Job there is described a mythical animal called behemoth. The word has come to denote any huge unassailable body. In so far as nurses are concerned, nurses in the aggregate, at any rate, the present-day behemoth is the modern hospital: a kind of immovable body to which nurses have yet to learn to apply an irresistible force.

Yet we in nursing can deal with the modern behemoth. We can assail it. We can tame it, if you will, and eventually turn it into a friend, a partner, with whom we can stride forward for the good of patients, for the good of our whole society. To do this, however, we must continue to keep clearly in mind at all times that our ultimate purpose is public service.

Over the years our record of public service has been excellent and it has been so recognized by the public. The criticism we receive today comes not from the public but from our own ranks and from hospital authorities. So far as the public is concerned, all that is wrong with nursing is that there aren't enough nurses. I believe that we have failed the public to some extent but the failure has been in public leadership, rather than in public service. Some authorities cite refusal to exercise public leadership as an indication of the "deprofessionalization" of a profession and they mention medicine and law as current examples. I suspect our failures have to do more with the struggle to actually become a profession and our inability to unite in sufficient strength to effect much leadership at all, much less public leadership.

That we are still struggling to become a profession is attested to by our unwillingness to unite in the interest of public service. There are 169,000 nurses in the American Nurses' Association. This sounds like a force for professional unity but the sad fact is that the ANA represents fewer than one third of the 550,000 nurses in practice in the United States. Unless the 169,000 can convince the foot-dragging 381,000 that our public service cannot continue to be rendered without a nursing profession united in sufficient strength to control its own practice, wherever that practice is performed, we shall have to wait for true professional status until the bulk of the 381,000 die off or retire from the ranks and are replaced by the less naive and the more thoughtful. By that time even the public will have caught on to the real reason for poor nursing care in hospitals. They will know by

Reprinted, with permission, from *The American Journal of Nursing*, LXV, January 1965, 77–78.

that time that the shortage of nurses is considerably less important than the failure of nurses to assume their responsibilities for nursing care. That the failure stems from ignorance rather than deliberate intent will not help much.

If none of this seems to have much to do with economic security, remember that economic security is not the primary purpose of the nursing profession. It is a means to an end, a very important means in today's society but a means nonetheless. Being a means rather than an end in itself in no way diminishes its necessity for us at our present stage of development as a profession. As a matter of fact, our conviction that it *is* a means to our primary purpose of public service should make the economic security program with its collective bargaining aspect more acceptable to the disdainful, the squeamish, the timid, the confused, and the naive.

Among the disdainful I would place some of our nursing leaders who, not now needing collective bargaining themselves, stand aloof from the whole process and mistakenly decry our lapse from the professional. It may well be that the lack of any organized effort toward economic security in their early days delayed their arrival as leaders much too long, to the detriment of themselves, the profession, and the public. They might ponder this and reflect on the relationship between low income and the development of nursing leaders or perhaps on the relationship between low income and apathy.

Among the squeamish and the timid I would place the many, many nurses who are entirely too sensitive to criticism from hospital and medical authorities without separating the constructive from the emotional and the double-dealing. For instance, we are told with monotonous regularity that nurses are no longer dedicated and we tend to cringe rather than to face squarely the question: Dedicated to what and to whom? Too many nurses, especially those in hospitals, are entirely too dedicated to some very old propositions that have no validity today and have too many misplaced loyalties. They are going to have to learn that patients and society have the first claim on their dedication and their loyalty. They are going to have to stop taking care of hospitals and doctors and give the best of themselves and their talents to patients and potential patients.

I am convinced that nurses do want to take care of patients. But without the conviction that nursing is theirs, without the conviction that they have rights and responsibilities upon which no other group may impinge, they cannot do much more than flounder. Nurses are beginning to have these convictions but, by and large, they are still ill prepared to fight for them.

Among the confused and the naive I would place all those nurses who say: "Of course we should have better salaries and better working conditions but the hospital doesn't have the money." Or, "Of course we should be able to give better care to our patients but there aren't enough nurses." Or perhaps, "Of course we should plan the nursing care of patients but the hospital system gets in the way." Or, "Of course we should be able to confer as a group with the hospital authorities but they say this is a union tactic and we shall lose our professional status."

All money for hospitals comes from the public, one way or another. How it is spent and why so much of it is needed is just becoming a public concern. We can hardly quarrel with hospital authorities for trying to hold the line, for trying to provide the best of everything for the lowest possible cost. Where we can and should quarrel with them is in the area of priorities. On the whole, hospital authorities have done an excellent job of producing the buildings that our new society seems to demand. They have equipped these institutions with the newest electronic devices, the most up-to-date scientific machines, and the most wonderful of the wonder drugs, no doubt with an eye on, but with little stickling at, the cost. They provide for doctors not only the workshops for modern medicine and surgery that the revolutionary changes in medical practice seem to require but also the freedom to use the workshops as they see fit. What is incredible is that they tend to think of nurses as a bulk payroll headache which prevents their keeping costs down. All too often we seem to accept this appraisal.

The ANA economic security program is designed to convince hospital authorities and nurses themselves that service is more important in a hospital than any type of material equipment, that the amount and quality of the service will be no better than the public is willing to pay for, and that the number of nurses available for hospitals even now, to say nothing of the future, depends on their recognition as a group of practitioners worthy of their hire.

As for that canard about our using union tactics, I am quite sure hospital administrators do not really believe this themselves. But it has been so effective you can hardly blame them for holding on to it. I suspect if we stopped cringing at the accusation, they would stop using it. We might try accusing them of restraint of trade or something similar. They refuse when they can to deal with us as a group but they have no compunction about getting together in a hospital council or a state hospital association to draw up a gentleman's agreement not to raise nurses' salaries and not to treat with state nurses' groups. Union tactics, indeed! We have learned them from the two professions we have always most admired. We have not yet learned, however, to utilize our majority status in hospitals or our scarcity as well as we might.

The issue at stake is not just better salaries, pensions, vacations, et cetera. The real issue is who shall control nursing, nursing practice, nursing quality.

At the moment, nursing pretty much is setting its own standards of practice but hospitals are dictating the performance of that practice. And the quality? It's a shambles! Nurses have permitted an erosion of both their rights and their responsibilities to result from their employment situation in the modern hospital. This is a failure in public service on the part of nurses at every level: the leaders who stand aloof; the academic nurses who are willing to wait for the next generation; the directors of diploma schools and of hospital nursing service departments who are unwilling to jeopardize their position with management; the rank and file who don't want to be bothered, who can't find any reserves of courage, who won't spend the money, who will not think. Sometimes I believe we are a sorry lot—but most of the time I think we just haven't learned how to loose the bonds of tradition while we maintain what is excellent in that tradition. Each of us hacks away a bit at the fetters but they will not be removed this way. We must think together; we must act together; we must unite in the public interest. Good care for patients and justice and freedom for nurses go hand in hand. Economic security for nurses is a means to an end. The end, public service, can no longer be attained without this particular means.

V PATIENT-CENTERED CARE

Concern for the welfare of the patient is both the oldest and newest focus in nursing. While nurses have always paid attention to the patient, this attention has been intensified and modified within recent years. Increasing concern has come to be centered on the problems of the patient and the abilities of nurses to search out the sources of these problems. To do this effectively the nurse has had to approach the patient with new questions and with new techniques. She has to determine what an illness means to a particular patient, and how she can help him cope with the problems associated with his sickness.

In emphasizing these new approaches to patient care, nursing is following developments in the behavioral sciences. Psychologists and psychiatrists have demonstrated that there are psychological problems associated with all kinds of illness, even those that seemingly are caused by purely physiological factors. Sociology has contributed to the change through the emphasis on the concept of the "sick role," namely, the assumption that the patient is faced with some necessary behavioral changes when he is ill, or when he must face the adjustment to a new handicap. (For the development of the concept of the sick role, see such works as Talcott Parsons and Renee Fox, "Illness, Therapy and the Modern Urban American Family," *Journal of Social Issues, VII,* 1952, pp. 31–44; Talcott Parsons, *The Social System,* Glencoe, Ill., The Free Press, 1951, especially chapter 10, and David Mechanic and Edmund Volkart, "Stress, Illness Behavior and the Sick Role," *American Sociological Review, XXVI,* Feb. 1961, pp. 51–58.) The very fact that sickness ordinarily excuses one from the normal obligations of every-day life causes problems; it necessitates learning a new role, that of the sick, in an unfamiliar setting, such as the hospital. It is often difficult for a patient to give up his status as a useful member of society and accept the dependency of the sick role.

Nursing itself has also contributed insights to this new patient-centered care. Pediatric nursing, in particular, has been an important area of change during the past decade, since long-term hospitalization of infants has become a common phenomenon. Even though new aseptic techniques and new treatments for formerly fatal diseases have drastically cut the mortality rate of hospitalized children from the almost 100 per cent of 1915, hospitalization of a child involves difficult nursing problems. (See René A. Spitz, "Hospitalism: An Inquiry into the Genesis of Psychiatric Conditions in Early Childhood," *The Psychoanalytic Study of the Child*, I. New York: International Universities Press, 1945, p. 53.) Researchers, such as René Spitz and William Goldfarb, (in Goldfarb's "Psychological Privation in Infancy and Subsequent Adjustment," *American Journal of Orthopsychiatry, XV*, 1945, 247–55), reported that infants who were confined to institutions of various kinds, including hospitals, developed a whole set of symptoms including listlessness, apathy, poor muscular coordination, and mental deterioriation. Even with scrupulous isolation techniques, the morbidity and mortality rates were higher for institutionalized infants than for those cared for at home. Goldfarb called this syndrome "psychological privation." Spitz at first called it "hospitalism" but later, as he noted the similarity to depressive illnesses, he termed it "anaclitic depression." (See René A. Spitz and Katherine M. Wolf, "Anaclitic Depression: A Inquiry into the Genesis of Psychiatric Conditions in Early Childhood." *The Psychoanalytic Study of the Child, II,* New York: International Universities Press, 1946, pp. 313–342.) Contemporary researchers, including the pediatric nurses whose papers are part of this section, call the syndrome "maternal deprivation." They suggest that it is a major nursing problem for those who care for hospitalized children.

Equally instrumental in bringing these new concepts to the attention of nurses were the psychiatric nurses who, by the nature of their specialty, are concerned with psychological problems. As psychiatric nursing developed, and as the mental hospitals shifted from custodial to treatment orientation, increasing attention was given to the role of the nurse in treatment. Since communication techniques became one of the most important occupational skills of psychiatric nurses, their newly developed methodology could be adapted to other areas of nursing.

Patient-centered care means different things in different settings. To understand the patient well in the medical or surgical ward is often to know that he needs a competent nurse, who will give him good physical care. To overlook this fact would be to turn "patient-centered" into a mere slogan rather than to make it a useful orientation. There exists as yet no clear-cut definition of what patient-centered nursing is, but, as the selections in this section indicate, the approach is being explored. There are many recent books that go into the various ramifications of patient-centered care. (*Newer Dimensions of Patient Care,* by Esther Lucile Brown, New York: Russel Sage Foundation, 1961, is one of the most important. See particularly Part I and Part III.)

Changes in the nurse's role have also contributed to this new emphasis. Much of what the nurse does is under the direction of the physician, but there is a growing realization on the part of nurse as well as physician, that there is an area of care which is really the domain of the nurse, including measures aimed at sustaining the patient and minimizing his discomfort. Given this area of relative autonomy, nurses are stimulated to do research to aid them in making more intelligent decisions. This research ranges in scope from the thoughtful questions of the individual nurse about her own work to the large-scale projects that employ sophisticated methodological tools. As research develops, it seems to be turning from peripheral issues toward its central focus, the patient. At the same time, the growing emphasis on research and academic achievement is recognized by nurses as a way of gaining status for their profession.

One of the persons who strongly urged nurses to pay more attention to the problems of patient care was Virginia Henderson. In an editorial for *Nursing Research* written in 1956, she urged that this important area of concern receive the attention it deserved.

32.
Research in Nursing Practice—When?

by Virginia Henderson

If research in any occupation were divided into two categories: 1) studies of the workers, and 2) studies of their work, which type would usually predominate? Would we find more research on lawyers or the law; on engineers or engineering; on cleaners or cleaning? In all these occupations, be they so-called "professions" or "vocations," the conclusion is the same—that there has been more research on practice than on the practitioner.

Reprinted, with permission, from *Nursing Research, IV,* February 1956, 99.

Why is it then, that in our field, studies on the nurse outnumber studies on the practice of nursing more than ten to one? (To define our terms, we should say here that we consider research on the nurse to include: studies of motivation, selection, and education of the nurse; needs and resources; the nurse's intellectual, social, and economic status, and her function or role in society; her satisfactions or dissatisfactions; her working and living conditions; the ways in which nurses are organized; and the laws affecting them. In contrast, studies on nursing practice are mainly concerned with the persons the nurse serves—the patient and his family—or at least with the equipment and materials used in giving the nursing care or treatment.

It can, of course, be argued that any study leading to improvement in recruitment, selection, preparation, and distribution of nurses; to better administration of nursing services; and to clarification of the nurse's role or function automatically affects practice. However, an even stronger argument might be made in the reverse—that research in the practice of nursing might even more substantially affect recruitment, role, status, preparation, needs, and working conditions.

Perhaps a wiser reaction to the undeniable fact that the bulk of nursing research deals with the worker rather than the work is to wonder why. Has society's demand for more and more nursing care made it necessary for the occupation to emphasize numbers, recruitment, and job satisfaction? Has the apprenticeship mold in which the nurse's preparation has been cast forced the occupation to confine its principle investigations to education of the nurse? Is the discrepancy between supply and demand responsible for the continuing studies of nursing resources, of patterns of nursing service, and of functional analyses in the major fields of nursing?

Another explanation of the focus of attention on the nurse rather than on nursing may lie in the sources of support received by nurses in advanced education where much of the research originates. University nursing programs, if not independent, are often associated with the university's school of education; sometimes the association is with the department of social sciences, occasionally with the department of biological and physical sciences, and in many cases with the schools of medicine. Is it possible that educators and social scientists have been more inclined to help nurses with their research than have the physical, biological, or medical scientists?

Do those in the latter categories tend to regard the nurse who participates in clinical research as a technician rather than as a partner, and have they discouraged the initiation of clinical research by the nurse? Is it also possible that it is easier to study the nurse than the patient? Is the study of the behavior of the sick so complex and so difficult that the research experts to whom nurses have turned for help been afraid of it? Or is it the nurse who shies away from studies that necessitate observation of the patient's reaction?

Another explanation of the paucity of clinical nursing research may lie in the pull of the well-prepared nurse toward administration or teaching. Since less than 10 percent of the "professional" nurses hold degrees of any kind, the supply of qualified administrators and teachers is inadequate to meet the demand. The well-educated nurse is pressured into teaching and administration, partly by the need for such services and partly by the fact that economic advancement and improvement of status are not generally available to the nurse who remains a practitioner. Clinical nurses whose collegiate training might prepare them to develop clinical research are rarely left to practice nursing.

It is not surprising that more than half of the 80 or more doctoral dissertations by nurses deal with education, and less than 15 percent with nursing care. The emphasis in master's theses follows somewhat the same pattern. Analyzing the contents of *Nursing Research* from 1952 to 1955 we note that more than half of the studies published relate to administration and education, while a little less than half relate solely or in part to clinical nursing. It is encouraging, on the other hand, to find some light thrown on a few basic nursing techniques, on health teaching, and on the patient's reaction to illness. In addition, interaction between nurses and patients is under investigation in many psychiatric hospitals. Judging by the number and excellence of such studies, it would seem that psychiatric nurses, more than those in any other field, are learning how to study nursing care.

Responsibility for designing its methods is often cited as an essential characteristic of a profession. Whether or not nurses achieve full professional status is unimportant, however, unless this development results in, or is accompanied by, improvement in nursing care in all its physiological and psycho-social aspects.

Nine years later, an unsigned editorial from *Nursing Outlook* (reprinted here in part) summarized the position and aims of nursing research and the development of a research attitude among nurses generally.

33.

Research Attitudes in Nursing

When research in nursing first began to take shape, the preponderance of the investigations centered on nurses themselves—their characteristics, their motivations, their public image, their frustrations and satisfactions, their relationships to each other, to physicians, to hospital administrators, and so on. The titles of the reports on these early projects attest to this. Perhaps this approach is the logical beginning for a profession to take, that is, to look at its members for a better definition of itself. Perhaps it is the kind of research with which the pioneers could be most comfortable. And maybe there was this inordinate emphasis on nurses, rather than on nursing, because much of the research in the early days was conducted or influenced by social scientists for whom the study of the behavior of nurses as a group held greater fascination than what nurses did. (Some day, a nurse researcher may find the study of social scientists as a group equally fascinating.)

As increasingly more nurses were trained in research methodology and as the body of knowledge specific to nursing research increased accordingly, research designed to test the theories basic to nursing practice began to emerge. And as nurses, generally, have become more sophisticated about research, they have lost their awe of it and have become less contented with their spectator role. For them, research is no longer the exclusive province of the few in the big league, contending that, as in baseball, sandlotters, little leaguers, bush leaguers, and minor leaguers are necessary adjuncts to a big league team. Nurses, generally, have begun to develop a research attitude.

Schools of nursing everywhere are studying their curriculums, teaching methods, and testing procedures. Some of them have been enabled by the Public Health Service, through its faculty research development program, to give their faculties an opportunity to acquire research skills, participate in research, and become more proficient in teaching research.

Hospitals and public health agencies throughout the country are engaged in a variety of studies to provide a sounder basis for improving services to patients than one that is constructed of adaptations to pressures and crises. The nursing practitioner is being challenged to test and evaluate her nursing care plans. The practitioners' findings and deductions may well be the key to full-scale research projects on the "why" of practices which we have accepted as gospel because we have always done them "that way."

Students in most schools of nursing are using the problem-solving approach to learning nursing content. Students in some of our baccalaureate programs are being taught how to use the abstractive process as an integral part of the

From an editorial. Reprinted, with permission, from *Nursing Outlook*, XIII, May 1965, 33.

development of nursing knowledge. Not all of these students on graduation will be researchers, but all will be vastly better prepared intellectually and psychologically than students of a decade or so ago to contribute to research and use its findings.

So much of what we have taught and practiced in nursing, and still do, has been based on tradition and empiricism. The development of action research should lessen our dependence on both. For this, we need the best research talent and consultation available, but mostly, we need teachers and practitioners who, in addition to being creative, have a research attitude.

> Two writers give their views on what illness is and what it means to the patients. Lederer in paper 34, outlines the stages of illness from the point of view of a psychiatrist, using the analogy of human developmental stages. In paper 35, Father van Kaam searches for the more subtle meanings from the point of view of an existentialist.

34.
How the Sick View Their World

by Henry D. Lederer

The experience of illness is a complex psychological situation. To clarify the responses of the sick to this experience it is necessary to consider three main time periods, each of which has a characteristic orientation.* These stages of the experience of illness are: 1) the transition period from health to illness, 2) the period of "accepted" illness and, 3) convalescence.

The Orientations of the Sick in the Transition Period from Health to Illness

Upon falling ill most persons become aware of undesirable, unpleasant, and painful sensations; of a disturbing reduction in strength and stamina; of a diminution in ability to perform habitual acts. For example, at the onset of an episode of virus pneumonia, the patient experiences headaches, vague chest pains, tightness of the skin. He fatigues easily, desires more than usual

---

* Barker, R. G., *et al.*, "Social psychology of acute illness," in *Adjustment to Physical Handicap and Illness* (rev. ed.). New York: Social Science Research Council, 1953.

From *Journal of Social Issues*, VIII, 1952, No. 4, 4–15.

rest, and "plays out" quickly on prolonged tasks. In addition he finds the performance of his daily routine of work and play tiring and aggravating to his discomforts.

One finds certain definite patterns of response to these initial events. Some degree of apprehension or anxiety is felt as in any situation in which a painful, unpleasant, and threatening circumstance is encountered.* Consequently the pattern of response to the initial symptoms is often the characteristic mode of reaction to anxiety whenever it arises. Many persons attempt to ignore this threat and through such a denial of the frightening experience to allay their anxieties. This denial may be reinforced by a "plunge into health" through engaging in more than routine activity. In this manner the patient seems to be reassuring himself by saying, "If I can manage to be so very active there is nothing to fear—the whole affair is an illusion." Another form of denial is to minimize the importance of the symptoms by identifying them with symptoms of benign or trivial indispositions. Thus the "coronary vascular accident" symptoms are identified with "an upset stomach" and the chest pains of lobar pneumonia with a "touch of pleurisy."

Still further, one observes other patients who meet anxiety aggressively and such persons in the initial stages of illness are irascible, querulous, and ill-humored. Conversely, others allay anxiety by passivity and behave in a compliant, obsequious, and pitiable manner.

The ordinary day-to-day life routines of most persons constitute a source of satisfaction of various needs and defenses against anxiety. Since illness renders painful and tiring participation in such gratifying and reassuring activities, anxiety is compounded and frustration of many needs is felt.** Thomas Mann has written humorously and understandingly of this experience in "The Magic Mountain." His hero, Hans Castorp, in the early febrile stage of an activated tuberculosis tries to preserve his daily rituals which have formerly proven gratifying and soothing. One of these practices is the smoking of the after dinner cigar, a luxury of great importance to Castorp; but now he finds an evil taste and light-headedness in the place of a delightful aroma and general feeling of well-being.***

Certain men become especially anxious when they find themselves having to restrict their activities and to admit the existence of their discomforts.**** To these persons, manliness depends on being active and never yielding to a physical discomfort; to them, passivity and any intolerance of pain are equated

* Binger, C. *The Doctor's Job.* New York: Norton, 1945.
** Upham, Frances, *A Dynamic Approach to Illness.* New York: Family Service Association of America, 1949.
*** Mann, Thomas, *The Magic Mountain.* New York: Knopf, 1945.
**** Barker *et al., op. cit.*

with femininity. Consequently, becoming ill is viewed as an emasculating process and, thereby, highly provocative of anxiety. There may be a danger-ous denial of symptoms in such a person through his abortive attempts to re-assert his masculinity in sports, late hours, heavy work, etc.

For many persons, parts of their bodies or certain bodily functions have been invested with intense emotion. The skin, the facial structures, the head, the genitals, the breasts are examples of bodily parts often intensely loved by the patient. Obviously great apprehension is experienced when symptoms seem to indicate dysfunction of these treasured parts.

There is a continuing folk tradition in some areas that suggests that illness is the just desert of the sinner. Persons holding to this misconception feel guilty when developing an illness and may even be impelled to malinger health rather than appear with the stigma of immorality.

Specific illnesses exhibiting a familial occurrence are particularly alarming since most persons do not want to discredit the purity of their families. This attitude has been one of the impedances to early diagnosis of such illnesses as carcinomata and tuberculosis. Often the afflicted person has great anxiety be-cause of the unconscious fantasy of rejection and wrath by the other members of the family. Most physicians have had contact with patients who are deeply shamed by symptoms which they interpret as a possible disgrace to their family lines.

Many persons, who, because of emotional immaturity and stressful living have been reduced to a psychoneurotic level of functioning, may react para-doxically to the advent of physical illness. Often there is an amelioration of the neurotic symptoms and the patient seems to welcome the concrete threat of physical illness which can divert his attention from his neurosis. With some neurotic persons, physical illness may actually bring emotional relief through its symbolic meaning as a penalty for unconscious guilt feelings. Moreover, the anticipated care and consideration as well as release from social responsi-bilities can be highly appealing to a neurotic patient. His feelings of guilt and shame for his withdrawing, dependent, and infantile wishes are relieved by the occurrence of physical sickness which "legitimizes" these claims. "The individual with a relatively weak ego may find an escape from his (neurotic) anxieties in the less demanding situation that illness provides.*

An example of this type of response to physical illness was observed in a young, single woman who was undergoing psychotherapy for severe phobias. Her neurosis developed in reaction to the stress of her approaching marriage for which her previous psychosocial growth had not prepared her. In the midst of this emotional distress, she developed visual and gait disturbances

* Upham, *op. cit.*

which were definitely diagnosed as symptoms of multiple sclerosis. At the onset of these grave symptoms and her entrance into hospital, she announced with elation that her phobic obsessions had departed and that she was entirely rid of anxiety.

To recapitulate, in the initial symptom phase of many illnesses, one may encounter evidence of anxiety, guilt, and shame as well as the many personality defenses against these disagreeable affects. Moreover, in certain neurotic patients there may be a paradoxically positive acceptance of illness.

The continuing pressure, and often the increase, of symptoms forces the patient into another psychologically difficult set of experiences—those of diagnosis and the beginning of therapy. At this time the former habitual patterns of health still exert a powerful attraction on the patient whereas his submission to diagnostic and therapeutic procedures involves entering an unknown area. But in order to be rid of his discomforts and dysfunctions he must face this unknown situation.

(It is important to note that at this point another crucial factor is met which influences the orientation of the patient—this factor is the behavior of the medical personnel who are responsible for his diagnosis and therapy.)

Whenever one enters an unknown or partially understood situation, he exhibits fairly typical responses. Once again anxiety is aroused because of fantasied dangers and because of unfamiliarity with what one may expect. Under these circumstances there is much indecision reflected in vacillating behavior. For example, urgent requests for diagnostic examinations are rapidly alternated with failure to appear for examination. Physicians must learn to expect such vacillating and indecisive behavior and not to be angered or disgusted by it. The firm, patient, and understanding attitude of the physician will help in allaying the patient's anxiety.

The highly scientific nature of medical diagnosis places these affairs beyond the full understanding of the average layman. The physical paraphernalia of many diagnostic processes are awesome to many persons. In addition, the technical language of medicine is an unknown tongue to the layman who can only hope that what he overhears is an optimistic statement rather than a pronouncement of doom or further pain for him. When these mystifying matters are coupled to the impersonality of diagnostic activity in many modern hospitals and clinics, it is easy to empathize with the mounting anxiety of the patient and his problem of cooperating in diagnosis.

• • •

When treatment requires a hospital setting, the doctor and his aides have the responsibility for explaining hospital procedures to the patient. The patient is able to cooperate more easily when he knows about such routine matters as the duty hours of the floor nurses, when meals are served, visiting rules, the names of his internes, etc. Often antagonistic, belligerent behavior can be charged to negligence in clarifying the hospital situation when the patient was admitted—it is his way of aggressively resolving his anxiety. The rate of "sign-out against medical advice" is inversely related to the success of the medical personnel in their handling of these problems.

The Stage of "Accepted" Illness

When the patient has accepted diagnostic and initial therapeutic procedures, he enters another distinct time period in his experience of illness. Now, he views himself as ill and abandons pretenses of health. In our society, accepting illness includes accepting help from physicians and their aides. He temporarily withdraws from his adult responsible activities and, cooperating with his doctor, dedicates himself to the problem of getting well; he substitutes preoccupation with his symptoms and illness for the many concerns of mature life. Whereas in health he has made his own decisions, he now transfers this right to his physician, nurse and other attendants. These changes in orientation are reinforced by the doctor's prescription that he not pursue his work, his usual recreations, nor his responsibilities. Society as a whole also frees him for the duration of his illness from the discharge of ordinary duties and obligations.

All of these changes determine the structure of the patient's world which can be described as a simpler, more childish, constricted life. His illness has led him into a social setting which is similar to his childhood.* Therefore, one can refer to this arrangement as being very regressed and infantile.

To such a regressed social situation the patient now reacts with behavior used earlier during his childhood. His actions, thoughts, and feelings are regressive in response to the child-like world of illness. The main features of this behavior are: 1) egocentricity, 2) constriction of interests, 3) emotional dependency, 4) hypochondriasis.**

Charles Lamb, in his essay, "The Convalescent," accurately described the egocentricity of the sick when he wrote, "How sickness enlarges the dimensions of a man's self to himself! he is his own exclusive object. Supreme selfishness is inculcated upon him as his only duty."*** Like a child the patient is concerned with the selfish matters of satisfying simple needs for rest, food, absence of pain, physical comfort, and relief of bodily tensions such as the urge to urinate, defecate, pass flatus, or to belch. Satisfaction of these needs assumes precedence over more social ones. The patient presumes

* Conference on Convalescent Care, New York Academy of Medicine, 1940.
** Barker *et al., op. cit.*
*** Lamb, Charles, *Essays.* New York: Viking, 1949.

that his attendants share in these preoccupations and he feels resentful or hurt if the doctor or nurse is distracted by other concerns.

His egocentricity renders him provincial and highly subjective, like a child, in his judging the events occurring around him. If the nurse frowns for a moment, he is worried that she has taken a dislike to him, if she does not respond to his ring, she is damned as lazy and uninterested in his welfare.

Often the patient becomes a sick-room tyrant, dominating others and intolerant or often unaware of their rights and needs. "If there be a regal solitude, it is a sick bed. How the patient lords it there"—"He keeps his sympathy, like some curious vintage, under trusty lock and key, for his own use only." This egocentric despotism frequently disturbs the friends and relatives of the patient who are accustomed to his former consideration and objectivity.

• • •

Dependence on others is imposed by the physical helplessness stemming from illness and by the psychological inadequacy secondary to egocentricity and constricted interests. The patient's physical weakness, like that of the child, requires the strength of other persons to meet his needs. His regression into a self-centered, subjective world demands that healthier persons apply their more mature and objective judgment to his affairs—again paralleling the experience of the child whose parents assume responsibility for most important matters. With this dependency, one observes much ambivalence toward the benefactors. Like a child the patient often exhibits an uncritical "love" and admiration for his benefactors, but at the same time resentment toward them because of his weak and inferior relation to them. All persons working with the sick should anticipate and learn to recognize this ambivalent dependency and neither be flattered, nor offended, by it.

The unpleasant sensations of illness, in combination with the reduced regressive world and perceptions of the patient, lead to a great concern with the functioning of the body. There is usually much hypochondriacal worry over medical matters such as pulse rate, temperature, bowel movements, weight changes, etc., all of which may dominate the patient's thoughts and conversations. This hypochondriasis resembles in some ways the curiosity and exploration of the body and its functions undertaken normally by all children.

The attitudes and behavior of the medical personnel can limit or extend the emotional regression of the patient. The appearance of apathy as a response to over-protection has already been cited.* In recent years, many

* Barraclough, W., "Mental reactions of normal children to physical illness," *American Journal of Psychiatry*, 1937, 93.

warnings have been sounded against unnecessary restriction of patients' activities.

The indiscriminate prescription of prolonged bed-rest has been demonstrated as a cause of invalidism out of proportion to actual physical incapacity. The current practice of encouraging patients to get on their feet as early as possible following operations has proven both physically and emotionally beneficial; it has prevented lengthy convalescence. It seems that the best course for the physician is to encourage the minimum amount of regression necessitated by the physical limitations of the patient and to avoid any unnecessary infantilizing.

This regression, during illness, is adaptive and often significant for survival. It is conceivable that through social and emotional regression the sick person re-distributes his energies to facilitate the healing process or possibly that the regressive integration is in itself an essential factor in the healing process. The biological task of the sick is to get well and this work is furthered by the focussing of personality energies on the self and withdrawing them from other uses and purposes.* Recognition of this utility in the regression of the sick should make medical attendants welcome it rather than deplore it.

In persons, whose general character development has led to elaborate behavior defenses against regression and the expression of dependency, there is little or no phase of "accepted illness." Denial of physical limits and symptoms continues to some extent; the advice and ministrations of medical personnel are challenged and not followed; hospital care may be refused. All in all the neurotic defenses of such a patient militate against the healing benefits of regression and the course of his illness may be worsened or fatal. His behavioral adjustment to his neurosis takes precedence over adaptive regression during physical illness.

To illustrate: A physician, in middle age, sustained an acute coronary heart attack. His professional colleagues, who diagnosed his illness, advised immediate and absolute bed rest, quiet, and heavy sedation, all of which the patient stoutly refused on the grounds of his heavy schedule of work with his own patients. He persisted in his medical work and died suddenly in his office twenty hours later. This patient's personality was structured largely to deny any dependent emotional trends. He was a "self-made" man who had labored hard to graduate from medical school. He steadfastly pursued his career, never permitting himself a vacation. In his personal life he lavished gifts on his family, but was Spartan in any self-indulgence. It can be conjectured that his neurotic character was a considerable factor in his early death.

* Ferenezi, S., "Disease or Patho-neurosis," in *Further Contributions to the Theory and Technique of Psychoanalysis*. London: Hogarth, 1926.

Under those conditions, the total medical management must include measures to aid the patient in accepting regression and dependency. At times a psychiatrist or psychiatric social worker must be included in the therapeutic team to contribute their skills in meeting this neurotic complication of a physical illness.

The period of "accepted illness" gradually ends after optimal regression and medical therapy have reversed or arrested the pathogenic process. The patient then enters the convalescent period of his experience of illness.

The Stage of Convalescence

Convalescence is the time period of transition from illness back into a state of health. This recovery of health involves a return of physical strength and a re-integration of the personality of the patient who has been living, feeling, and thinking in a regressed, more or less infantile way.

The return of physical strength and health is usually an automatic process but it is not necessarily paralleled by a restoration of "healthy," adult behavior; getting well physically must be associated with the patient's relinquishing his dependent, egocentric and provincial reactions.*

Many students of convalescence have recognized its structural and dynamic similarities to adolescence. This analogy is instructive in understanding the problems of the convalescent and suggests many techniques for helping the convalescent "grow up" again into adult health.**

The convalescent, like the adolescent, has to leave a protected world in which responsibilities were minimal and the satisfaction of his self-centered needs the major concern of himself and those attending him. These pleasant aspects of illness attract the convalescent so that he wants to remain in his "regal home" of regression. It is hard for one to give up the attentions, protection, and kindnesses of doctors and nurses and to fend once more for oneself. "Farewell with him all that made sickness pompous—the spell that hushed the household—the mute attendance—the inquiry by looks—the still softer delicacies of self-attention—what a speck is he dwindled into [by his physical recuperation]."***

If the patient has suppressed his resentful hostility toward his medical attendants during the preceding phase, he frequently remains regressed because of a guilty over-dependence upon them. Recent studies on poliomyelitis patients who require respirators have shown that the patients who are slowly

---

* Romano, J., "Emotional components of illness," *Connecticut State Medical Journal,* 1943, 7.
** Baker, *et al., op. cit.*
*** Lamb, *op. cit.*

"weaned" from the "artificial lung" are those who have been unable to express openly any negative feelings toward their doctors and nurses.*

Convalescence is often prolonged in persons whose previous state of health did not provide them with sufficient gratifications and relief from anxiety. Examples of this situation are seen in military service where full recovery from illness means re-entering a hazardous and depriving existence.

Fortunately, for most convalescents, the broader scope of their "healthy" worlds is more attractive than the regressive pleasures of illness. In such persons the stronger motive is toward health but may be impeded by continuing feelings of inadequacy. Like adolescents who yearn for adult life but feel unsure of themselves, these convalescents wistfully long for health but are afraid to try it. These fears may be related to neurotic self-depreciation which was part of the original behavior pattern in childhood, reactivated during the period of regression.

Certain convalescents repeat their adolescent method of "growing up" by rebelliously wrenching themselves loose from dependency. These persons are in a tremendous hurry to get well, often prematurely dismiss their physicians, and over-step their physical strengths.

Again one realizes that the participation of the physician and his aides can profoundly affect the course of convalescence. Under these conditions the medical personnel occupy roles similar to those of the parents and counselors of adolescents; the successful medical management of convalescence is the analogue of proper parenthood during adolescence.

To illustrate: The parent who gradually and progressively relaxes his protection and instead offers guidance and advice is encouraging the adolescent toward adulthood. He quietly retires to the side-lines ready to reassure but willing to let his child experiment with new strengths, only stepping in when gross errors of judgment may arise. The adolescent senses the confidence of the parent and is reassured by it, especially when immediately perfect or ideal results are not demanded. Moreover, the helpful parent is not threatened by his child's interest in other persons or new activities.

Convalescence can be promoted and enhanced by similar attitudes on the part of the doctor. Physicians must have the courage to recommend more activity and to lift the restrictions on the patient's behavior. Some physicians, like parents, are unconsciously gratified by the dependency of others upon them; this narcissistic pleasure must be abandoned by no longer encouraging regressive dependency through protection. The physician sometimes is loath to risk his reputation through the possibility of a relapse and thereby continues to treat the convalescent with great caution; this is frequently the

* Unpublished data from studies in progress, Department of Psychiatry, College of Medicine, University of Cincinnati.

event when the patient is a person of some prominence in the community so that his illness has been under a public scrutiny which makes the physician uneasy.

The rehabilitation of the convalescent has become a matter of growing medical concern, research, and progress. During the war the military medical services were alert to these problems and contributed many important findings to this aspect of medical management.* Since the war some of the medical colleges have established departments of rehabilitation as integral basic training units.

Offering the convalescent stimulation for re-integration is stressed. Increasing visiting privileges, permitting the wearing of ordinary rather than hospital clothes, providing radio and television, permitting trial leaves overnight from the hospital are examples of opportunities which may stimulate the patient toward a state of health. Transfering the convalescent to a special rehabilitation center or ward has been recommended as an aid in helping him relinquish the regressive patterns of life followed on ordinary hospital wards.

The modern physician is urged to lead a team of therapists in the guidance and support of the convalescent just as the wise parent welcomes the contributions of the teacher, youth leader, student counselor, etc. who promote the growth of the adolescent. Social workers, occupational therapists, vocational counselors, recreational therapists, etc. can broaden the scope of the convalescent's world, encourage him and help re-establish his self-confidence and self-sufficiency.

While the patient is still in the state of "accepted illness," the caseworker may have discovered sources of tension and dissatisfaction in his family, home, or work situations and can initiate changes which will make the return to health more attractive. In addition the cooperation of the family in the management of convalescence is often won by a skillful caseworker.

Much attention has been given to occupational therapy through which the patient is gently led into a more self-assertive, creative life. Moreover, he is given the opportunity to re-exercise rusty talents and techniques in an experimental setting. Here he can regain self-confidence through a series of progressive "successes."

Well-planned recreational therapies provide practice in socializing and in engaging in gradual competition. Here again the success in group living encourages the patient to re-enter the large arena of adult "healthy" society.

* Watson-Jones, R., "Rehabilitation in the Royal Air Force," *British Medical Journal*, 1942, 1, 403–407; Wilson, E. H., "Rehabilitation in war-time Britain," *Archives of Surgery*, 1943, 46; and Thorndike, A., "Convalescent reconditioning, *American Medical Association Journal*, 1944, 126.

The expanding use of vocational counseling is an indication of its value to the convalescent. Many patients cling to regressed behavior because they cannot engage further in past occupations. For example, convalescent tuberculous patients frequently must find less strenuous jobs to protect them from relapses. In such a situation, hopeful and realistic planning can be constructed through consultations with a competent vocational counselor. The convalescent, like the adolescent, is less afraid of his future when his vocational potentialities are clear to him.

In addition to the special services each member of the therapeutic team has to offer, there is the over-all benefit of providing the patient contact with many mature, healthy persons with whom he can emotionally identify. This process is similar to the identification of the adolescent with key adult persons in his environment. Both the convalescent and adolescent find such identification a most positive aid in accepting an adult status. Conversely, emotionally immature persons serving on therapeutic teams can seriously retard the convalescent's recovery by not providing the bridge of a healthy identification.

All of these various services and stimuli can be offered to a patient but it is necessary to realize, no one can force him to use them constructively. For the majority of persons "health" is preferred to regression. With the few patients who cannot respond positively to planned convalescence, one usually finds that an earlier neurosis has been revived by the trauma of illness; these persons should be offered psychotherapy to resolve the neurotic difficulties prolonging their full recovery.

To summarize: the state of convalescence is structurally and dynamically similar to adolescence. The behavior of the convalescent is analogous to that of the adolescent. The success of helping the patient is dependent on the recognition of his "adolescent" emotional status which then should call forth from his medical attendants attitudes similar to those of the parent who encourages and aids the growth of his adolescent child. Opportunities must be provided for re-establishing self-confidence through graded "successes" in groups and in the exercise of one's returning physical strengths. The convalescent phase of illness terminates with the parallel recovery from physical limitation and psychological regression.

35.

The Nurse in the Patient's World

by Adrian L. van Kaam

In order to become more deeply aware of what it means to be sick, let us consider in a very condensed form, an analysis of the experience of a person who is sick. This analysis is based on descriptions given by the Dutch psychiatrist, J. H. van den Berg, and by the French author, France Pastorelli.

Probably every one of us has undergone illness and may try to remember what happened to him. When you cannot leave your bed in the morning you hear outside your room the noises of the house, the children, the kitchen. The sounds in your house are the same and still they are different. You hear people leaving the house. Out there is the usual beginning of your daily life. But you feel as an outsider who does not participate, who does not have a function in it. There seems to be a distance between you here in this bed and those familiar sounds.

Somebody before leaving will come up to your room and ask how you are feeling. His brief presence makes the distance still greater and deeper. Everything about your visitor tells you about the usual healthy day, the day of work, of play, of the street and of the school, of the day outside your room, your house. But today this outside takes on a new meaning in your life.

The new day started also in the street under your window. There is the shouting of boys, the noise of the cars, the sudden screaming of brakes. But again you feel as an outsider, and the street and the polyphony of sounds otherwise so familiar to you seem strange now and at a distance. During the day the telephone rings, the doorbell rings, but you no longer participate. The world seems to be reduced to this sick room, to this bed.

As soon as you step out of bed and into the room, it is as if you were entering unknown territory, it is like leaving your house. When you go to wash your hands, you experience it more or less as an unreal excursion. Back in your bed you have the feeling of being home again.

The plans of yesterday are losing their importance, the future is losing its attraction. The contours of the future are becoming blurred. You retire into the small limited now. You live only the moment of this bed, which protects you against what is and what is to come. When you are healthy you live mostly in the future and you forget the moment in your reaching out to what comes next. But now, being sick, you are not able to escape this moment.

Reprinted, with permission, from *The American Journal of Nursing*, LIX, 1959, 1708–1710. (Extract).

Another experience is your heightened awareness of your body. When you are healthy you usually forget about your body as you do your work. But when you are sick, your body announces itself loudly and obtrusively in a headache, a vague nausea. The body of which you were mostly unaware becomes now the center of your attention. As a sick person you live with a body that seems not useful but a nuisance.

Another change occurs. Many things around you assume a meaning which they did not have as long as you were healthy. The usual ring of the telephone becomes a new kind of sound in a house which is remarkably strange and distant. You never noticed before the color of the blankets on your bed; now they look like woods of hairy colored threads. The sheets become white plains with clefts, hills, and mountain tops. And you catch yourself analyzing the wallpaper into stripes, points and figures.

The changes are still deeper in a serious sickness. Every year thousands of people discover that they have cancer, or are disabled, or are paralyzed by a series of strokes or a sudden accident. At this discovery their daily world seems to collapse. They no longer have an eye for their cherished possessions and their ambitious projects. They may even see the people around them in a different light. They feel that they are in another class of people—the sick—while others belong to the caste of the healthy.

The beginning of serious sickness is a stop, a break, a being cut off. Life seems to fade out for a while. Then another kind of life takes over. But the patient cannot know of the new values that can become his in this new way of life. He is suspicious and fearful of the unknown that looms up for him after the crude and sudden destruction of his familiar daily routine. He is afraid of the loneliness, the weakness, the suffering and pain which await him.

He thinks that the values implied in the life of a sick person are so small and insignificant that they will not be able to give form, shape, and substance to a life that seems lost and empty. He feels darkly and vaguely that one is not really able to "live" this new strange life. It seems to him that he may only be able to endure it, defeated, crushed, bewildered, perplexed, rebellious, or in fruitless passive resignation.

Because he is overwhelmed by this new experience, everything becomes uncertain for him. He is uncertain about his personal function in the life of others, about the necessity or even indispensability of his existence. He feels uncertain of the future and he loses confidence in the integrity of his body which has betrayed him so cruelly.

And, paradoxically, precisely because access to the world is blocked, life becomes more attractive and beautiful than it ever was before. Once the patient discovers that he is incurable and on his lonely way to death, the world seems to flow way from him, he feels isolated from life and the universe, but at the same time the world assumes a warm familiarity, a glow unknown in the noisy past. Every little thing—a flower, the smile of a child, the color of a falling leaf—exudes an intensity, an excitement not discovered before in the hustle and bustle of daily life. They evoke feelings that are sweet and painful. The certainty of death makes life livelier than ever before. This is a surprising experience which never disappears completely during the long months of sickness.

Then, another drama sets in. France Pastorelli calls it "le drame avec l'entourage." It is the hidden conflict between the sick person and his visitors, due to the deep chasm between the way in which the visitor sees the sick and the way in which the sickness is lived by the patient himself.

The sick person never overcomes completely the surprise he felt at becoming sick. Even the serious illness, prolonged over many years, is never experienced by the patient as an indisputable fact, a closed door. So the sickness retains some of its surprise for the patient himself but, as time goes on, he no longer detects surprise on the face of the friend who visits him. He is asked how he feels but when he answers, he senses that his friend's mind is occupied with other things going on in a world in which he does not seem to belong any longer. His visitor displays tactfulness. This very display emphasizes for the patient that he is different, that he has become someone with whom one has to deal in a very delicate way.

The sick person cannot communicate with his visitor about this new kind of life—this lonely facing of sickness and death. Modern man has repressed the thought of these unpleasant realities, and society cooperates by removing their signs from the public scene, which is dominated by the cult of the radiant health. Modern man is an awkward visitor to the sick because he does not know how to converse about sickness and death. He feels relieved when he is back in his car among the familiar sounds and sights of the street.

On the other hand, the sick person who does not cling grimly to his past but who accepts his new situation will discover a new life of surprising intensity. He will become sensitive to the great manifestation of being in the small things surrounding him. The sick person knows as no other the rhythm of the day: how his window catches the first hesitating light in the early morning, the playful spots of mild sunlight in his room hours later, the long and lazy noon, the quiet approach of the evening, the stillness and the darkness of an endless night. All of these things may not necessarily become agreeable to the patient, but they gain a new intimacy and familiarity. He can be fascinated by the opening of a flower in the window frame, the travels of a fly on the lampshade, a passing bird, a dog barking in the street.

This is a summary of only certain aspects of the existence of the sick.

It may serve as a guide for the nurse who tries to understand the patient as a sick person, but she must make a further effort to understand him as an individual.

In order to discover what it means to feel understood by a person, we performed existential research, studying 365 subjects. The following definition is based on the results of that research, applied to the nurse-patient relationship.

That a patient feels really understood by a nurse means that *the patient perceives that the nurse as a person co-experiences what things mean to him and still accepts him. As a result of this, the patient initially feels relief from his experiential loneliness and, gradually, begins to feel safe experiential communion with this nurse and with that which he perceives her to represent.*

In this descriptive definition, the patient perceives that the nurse co-experiences with him his new and frightening world. His feeling of really being understood, however, depends on his being able to sense her understanding. The nurse has to show in her attitude, her behavior, her whole personality that she understands the patient. The patient has to perceive the nurse as a person, a fellow human being, not as a technician exclusively. When we say that the understanding nurse "co-experiences" we mean that she not only knows or perceives or comprehends, for instance, that the patient is afraid of surgery, but as a human being she shares with him the experience of fear.

The patient in our descriptive definition who feels understood perceives that the nurse understands what things mean to him. We could describe this perception as follows: the patient perceives that the understanding nurse experiences the events, situations, and behavior which affect him, not in the way that they might affect *her* but in the way that they affect *him*.

The content of the words "still accepts him" in the definition can be summarized: the patient perceives that the understanding nurse, while co-experiencing his views, feelings, and behavior, even those which she cannot wholly accept personally, manifests consistently genuine interest, care, and basic trust in him. This she does whether or not the patient intends to change his views, feelings, or behavior.

According to this description, the nurse's manifestation of interest, care, and trust must be consistent. The patient who looks for understanding is extremely sensitive to even the slightest sign of disapproval, rejection, condemnation, or lack of interest. Her interest has to be perceived as genuine and honest; it cannot be feigned. Patients in their intensified sensitivity distinguish sharply between genuine and pretended interest, care, and trust.

The term "interest" emphasizes the undivided sympathetic attention of the understanding nurse. "Care" means that the patient perceives that the understanding nurse really has his well-being at heart, that she does not pursue her own selfish purposes. "Basic trust" means that the nurse believes in the real but perhaps hidden potentialities in the patient for accepting and overcoming his problems. The patient perceives that this faith of the nurse in his possibilities for good cannot be destroyed by anything she sees in him.

The nurse can accept this person in spite of the fact that his views or behavior are not personally acceptable to her. She can accept him because she recognizes in all his views, feelings, and behavior a wrestling, suffering, now victorious, now defeated human person who is trying to come to terms with illness.

When we study the feelings of the patient who feels really understood, we discover among them the feeling of relief at being understood in this new lonely world. The patient is alone, suddenly cut off from his former way of life. But his feeling of loneliness recedes to the degree that he experiences real understanding.

Gradually the nurse and all that she really or symbolically represents for the patient—the doctors, the hospital, the treatments, that whole mysterious universe of being sick—become less frightening. The communion of experience he feels with the nurse helps the patient to converse with all the new things which are entering his life. He feels more and more safe because he is sharing his experience.

Through his communion with "the nurse" as both a real and symbolic aspect of the world of the sick, the patient can gradually face the other aspects of his new existence without crippling anxiety or aversion.

Obviously the nurse plays a significant role in her relationship with the patient. Patients tend to invest the nurse with special emotional and symbolic meaning. In effect, the nurse becomes involved in the private world of each patient, often without quite realizing what the patient expects of her, or without recognizing that the patient's requests and complaints may have little or no relation to the actual care and treatment he needs. A patient may receive care of high professional quality, yet he may neither know nor be concerned about it because he is occupied with the drama of his private world wherein physicians, nurses, orderlies, and other medical figures become symbols or surrogates for the significant persons in his life experience. A major task for the nurse is to understand the patient's problems as well as she can, and to use her relationship with him to aid in his recovery. In papers 36 and 37 the nurse-patient relationship is discussed.

36.

Understanding the Nurse-Patient Relationship

by Thelma Ingles

Two small studies have been done recently by students at Duke University School of Nursing in Durham, North Carolina, which are pertinent to the understanding of the nurse-patient relationship.

The first study was done by a graduate student during her clinical practice in the hospital. Because she observed that nurses labeled patients as "good" or "bad," she began to wonder what characteristics of patient behavior elicited these labels. In investigating the characteristics, she asked a sample of some 60 nurses in two hospitals to describe the most common characteristics which influence judging a patient as good or bad. Her sample included both graduates of diploma and university programs, and a small number of junior basic students. The replies were categorized by a committee consisting of herself, a clinical psychologist, a sociologist, and a nurse faculty member.

In rank order, the "good" patient was judged good because he possessed the following characteristics: noncomplaining, nondemanding, cooperative with doctor's orders, appreciative of staff, helps self, and physically and conversationally pleasing.

The characteristics of the "bad" patient in rank order were: demanding, complaining, physically and conversationally displeasing, does not help self, unappreciative, and uncooperative. Although the rank order changed, the bad patient was perceived as having characteristics opposite from those of the good patient. Also, four of these characteristics can be interpreted as reflecting both the pressures and tensions and the reward systems of hospitals.

Patients who are noncomplaining, nondemanding, cooperating with doctor's orders, and who help themselves require less of the nurse's time and energy than do complaining, demanding, uncooperative patients who refuse to help themselves. Good patients permit nurses to get their tasks finished. Nurses who get their tasks finished in a proper fashion are perceived as good nurses, and are commended. There is a reality factor here: beds must be made, baths given, pills distributed, and treatments done. These are the things which can be recorded as completed—the tangibles of nursing care. They do not require that nurses become involved in patient behavior, in the qualitative aspects of the nurse-patient relationship—in the behavior of the nurse with a patient, or the behavior of a patient with a nurse.

What is the significance of a complaint and a demand? A complaint may be defined as a dissatisfaction, a wish for a change in the way things are. If a

Reprinted, with permission, from *Nursing Outlook*, IX, 1961, 698–700.

complaint is not met and handled to the satisfaction of the patient, it becomes a grievance, and grievances result in demands. Thus, if a patient wishes to be labeled good, he must not complain. He must accept his illness with all of its personal threats, the discomforts of unpleasant and frightening symptoms, the uncertainties of diagnostic and therapeutic procedures; he must accept these and remain silent. If he rebels against the problems created by his illness and complains, he will be judged a bad patient. If his complaints become demands, he will be judged "worst of all."

Why do patients complain? The source of a patient's complaint may be overt, easily observed, interpreted, and handled. The baby may fuss or scream because his diaper is wet and he feels uncomfortable. A dry diaper may then make him more comfortable and end his fussing.

On the other hand, the source of a complaint may be covert, disguised. The baby with a wet diaper may be crying not because of the wetness of his diaper, but because he thinks it is about time for someone to pay attention to him. The changing of the diaper may then relieve either physical or psychic discomfort.

I remember a very special aide, Nellie, who had the facility for interpreting intuitively the needs of babies. When the ward became particularly upset by the vocal complaints of many babies, the supervisor would send for Nellie. When Nellie arrived, she would survey the situation and simply start at one end of the ward and work through to the opposite end. She would look at a screaming baby, make a diagnosis, and act appropriately. For one, she changed his diaper; for another, she picked him up, patted him, comforted him, and returned him quietly to his bed. For another, she got a bottle of water; for another, a toy. She saw a baby's need, fulfilled it, and passed on to the next baby. I don't think she ever saw a baby as either good or bad, but simply as one needing something from her.

On one occasion, I remember watching Nellie as she stood in a doorway looking at a young student trying to feed a baby. The baby, with every muscle taut, was screaming at the top of his lungs. The student was frantically trying to get the nipple into his rebellious mouth. Finally, Nellie could stand it no longer. She walked over, took the baby from the student, held him tightly for a moment, sat down, presented the bottle to him, and he gratefully accepted it. Nellie said to the student, consolingly, "Honey, this baby knew you were scared of him and he knew you were mad at him. That is why he wouldn't eat. You don't ever have to be scared of babies, or mad at them. They are pretty little."

I also remember with pleasure a practical nurse who had this same intuitive capacity for recognizing and meeting patients' needs. I first met this practical nurse in a class in which one of my students was practice teaching. The class was on child behavior, and the practice teacher began by saying to the group, "Many of you have children. Have any of you had any problems with your children which you would like to tell us about?" One of the students said, "I'd like to tell you about a problem I am having with my little boy right now. He wants to eat with a fork like his Daddy does. Now, I think he is too little to eat with a fork; forks are dangerous. But, he is too little to understand this, and at every meal we have trouble."

The practice teacher accepted this as a real problem, and asked the class if they had any suggestions. One of the students raised her hand and stated simply, "I know what I would do if he were my little boy. I'd make his Daddy eat with a spoon. In a few days he wouldn't care whether he had a spoon or a fork." This practical nurse did not see the child as bad because he wanted to eat like his Daddy. She looked at the situation, and out of her intuitive understanding of children, identified the problem and came up with a reasonable and workable solution.

Sometimes the patient hides a real complaint with superficial ones. One patient, Mrs. Black, had been in our hospital several times for treatment of acute phases of multiple sclerosis. She had always been a very cheerful, noncomplaining patient, beloved by the ward staff. During this particular hospitalization, however, she was an irritable, unhappy, complaining, and demanding patient. She complained about all the details of her care—about her diet, her messy room, about having to wait, about not being cared for properly. Her change in character was strange to the doctors and nurses on the ward, and they seemed to resent it. Her staff physician asked me if I would have one of the students talk with her because he felt there was something bothering her which we didn't understand.

I asked one of my students to talk with her. She saw her for a few minutes that morning just to get acquainted. In the afternoon she returned for twenty minutes, rubbed her back, and made her as comfortable as possible. The next day she spent about two hours with her, giving her morning care. The student asked no questions, but was quiet and loving in her care. After she began bathing her, Mrs. Black began to talk about her mother who had lived with her and her family for two years. Her mother had a serious cerebral accident which left her severely handicapped. During the last month of her illness she was incontinent. Mrs. Black's tone of voice told the student that caring for her incontinent mother had been extremely difficult for her. She talked about the number of times she had had to change the bed, about the odors in the room which had seemed to invade the whole house, about the feelings of her husband and her two daughters toward her mother. She even described her own guilt in feeling as she did toward her mother. When Mrs. Black finished she seemed very depressed and was quiet. After a while she said, "I have been incontinent twice this past month. I can't bear to have my family feel toward me as we did toward my mother."

This illustrates how a patient may verbalize multiple complaints, yet not speak of the real complaint. Mrs. Black didn't really care about the diet, her messy room, or having to wait. These were simply safe complaints. She was so frightened of her real complaint that she couldn't talk about it. But we couldn't help her until we identified her real complaint.

In many instances an interested and sensitive person can intuitively help in the solution of a problem. In Mrs. Black's situation, more than intuition was necessary. She required a nurse who could accept and tolerate her little complaints; a nurse who could behave in a particular way, in a way which made it possible for her to feel safe and comfortable in relating her fears; a nurse who could listen through, who by verbal and nonverbal ways could help her talk. Mrs. Black needed a nurse who had the sensitivity to recognize the significance and the meaning of incontinence to Mrs. Black.

It seems quite apparent, then, that a patient's complaint is often a plea for help, an expression of a need for a certain kind of behavior from the nurse. The source of the complaint may derive from a simple need, such as a glass of water, or it may derive from a more diffuse need, such as anxiety relative to a prognosis.

The ways by which a nurse responds to a patient's complaint also vary in their derivation; they may derive from feelings relative to a specific complaint, a particular patient, or from feelings which are actually remote from either the specific complaint or the patient. A patient may complain loudly that his bowels have not moved for two days. In a hospital, many patients complain about constipation. The very subject, when brought up by a patient, may irritate the nurse to the point where she will respond with a tone of voice which shows indifference, or even disgust. As a result of this verbal gesture, the patient may react by feeling "nobody cares about me," and become depressed; or he may become a demanding patient.

A nurse who grew up with a very autocratic and rigid grandmother may interpret even the minor complaints of an elderly woman as bossiness, and without understanding her own feelings, label the old lady as a bad patient. I remember one old lady who was a patient in our hospital. This old lady had dipped snuff for 60 or 70 years, and continued this untidy habit in the hospital. The nurse assigned to care for her had a very strong aversion to sputum, and as a result condemned this old lady's every gesture and comment. The old lady could do nothing right. One day, the nurse could stand it no longer, and tried to persuade her to give up this disgusting habit. The old lady turned to her and said quietly, "Why, ma'am, if it weren't for snuff, there wouldn't be any Duke Hospital."

Feelings which are remote from either the complaint or the patient are the feelings which the nurse may bring with her to the patient, and for which the patient has no "responsibility." For example, if a nurse has had a fight with her boy friend, has failed an examination, has been scolded by a head nurse or a doctor, her level of irritability may be raised to the point where she will interpret even a simple comment as a complaint. She may displace her feelings, generated by her previous problem, onto the patient, and in effect say, "You keep still. I have plenty of my own problems to worry about."

In any nurse-patient relationship, the nurse needs to look at herself as well as at the patient. She needs to develop self-awareness, and awareness of how she sees specific complaints and complaints in general; an awareness of how she perceives individual patients and patients in general; an awareness of how she feels in a particular place at a particular time. Does she behave differently with old patients and young patients, men and women, rich and poor, illiterate and well-educated, Negro and white, docile and aggressive, quiet and talkative, grateful and ungrateful, Catholic and Protestant, believers and nonbelievers?

Furthermore, she must become aware of herself, and understand her own feelings when she meets her expectations and when she does not meet her expectations. She must become aware of the extent to which she inflicts her self-expectations on others. If she demands orderliness of herself, does she demand this in others, too? If she demands courtesy in her own actions, does she demand courtesy in others? If she expects to meet all the vicissitudes of life with courage and fortitude, does she expect this same strength of others?

I remember walking through the hospital corridor outside the operating room and coming upon a small boy sitting upright in his crib with a look of sheer panic on his face. I walked over to him and said, "What's the trouble, fellow?" With an outburst of feeling he said, "The nurses say I have to be brave, and I don't want to be brave." I picked him up and said, "You don't have to be brave if you don't want to be brave." He cried, because he wanted and needed to cry. I stayed with him until it was his turn to go in for surgery. Then I walked back to his ward and said to his nurse, "Why did you leave that little boy outside of the operating room to wait alone?" She said, "This is the twenty-seventh time he has gone to the operating room for surgery. He knows what it is all about." I replied, "I think he had 27 reasons for being scared."

This nurse expected this little boy to face the ordeal of surgery as she thought she would expect to face it herself, or perhaps as she had once been expected to face it. She failed to understand or accept the fact that this little boy just couldn't be brave enough to face alone his twenty-seventh experience with surgery.

In a relationship with a patient, then, it is important for the nurse to understand herself before she tries to understand patients. What are her needs, her aspirations, her expectations? Only through self-understanding can a nurse become objective in her care of patients. By developing objectivity, she can respond to patients' needs rather than expect them to respond to hers. By being objective, she will be able not only to permit a patient to be hostile, but able also to encourage him to be hostile because she understands that "cloistered hostility" may play havoc with a patient's soma. So, perhaps, in the beginning of any relationship, the nurse should ask herself, "How do I really feel toward this patient, about this patient? What does he do or say that pleases or displeases me? Why does it please or displease me?" Only through understanding her own feelings can the nurse tolerate and cope with the feelings of patients.

Another study at Duke was concerned with the nurse-patient relationship. This study was done by a senior basic student who was interested in the effects of a patient's hostility on ward staff, and of the ward staff's hostility on a patient. She wondered if it would be possible to change the behavior of one by changing the behavior of the other. She elected to try to help patients change their behavior.

This student used our private medical wards for her sample, and studied a total of 14 patients. In the afternoon she would ask the head nurse on one of the wards for the name of the most difficult patient on the ward. She also asked staff nurses, student nurses, and auxiliary workers. After selecting the "winner" for the most difficult position, she asked permission to care for this patient the following morning. She gave the patient four hours of care, from 8:00 A.M. until 12 noon. During these four hours she attempted to be the kind of nurse the patient wanted and seemed to need.

The following morning she returned to the ward and casually asked the staff for a report on the patient's behavior. "How has Mr. A been behaving?" For each of the 14 patients she studied, the ward reported an improvement in the patient's behavior. Complaints were fewer, lights were on less often, and the ward staff seemed to perceive each patient with less hostility.

I would like to see this study repeated with a larger sample, and also for the purpose of testing long-term results. I predict that if you could change a patient's behavior so that the ward perceived him with less hostility, the staff's behavior with him would change, and, as a consequence, the patient would receive better care. As he received better care, he would have less need to be hostile.

The behavior of the nurse with a patient is an integral part of the patient's therapy. A positive nurse-patient relationship is good for the patient. Today we have more than humane reasons for finding this true. Research in psychosomatic medicine has produced abundant evidence that stress produces undesirable effects on the body. Stress may elevate a patient's blood pressure, an undesirable effect for the hypertensive patient. Stress may elevate the blood sugar, an undesirable effect for the diabetic patient; stress may increase the motility of the stomach, an undesirable effect for the patient with gastric ulcers. Certainly the nurse cannot remove all of the patient's reactions to the stresses of living which he brings with him to the hospital. She can, however, modify some of the stresses of hospitalization, and help him tolerate better those which she cannot modify. A good emotional experience in the hospital may then give him strength to cope with the problems he will face when he goes home.

A positive nurse-patient relationship is good not only for the patient, it is good for the nurse. There can be no greater satisfaction for the nurse than the knowledge that through her personal ministrations she has helped a patient feel better. Nursing, perhaps more than any other profession or occupation, permits its members to be loving and tender, to reach out to another with sincere warmth and compassion. One of the wonderful things about being a nurse is that the nurse can give of herself to another without feeling embarrassed or inhibited. She doesn't have to be afraid to be kind.

37.
Clarifying Patients' Communications
by Mary C. Dye

Can a nurse safely assume she has relieved a patient's distress without asking him how he feels about what she has done? Do patients' requests and comments always indicate clearly what they need?

The following example is taken from a study initiated by this writer, designed to help find the answers to these and other similar questions.

Around 2:00 o'clock one afternoon a surgical patient started pacing in front of the nurses' station.

"Where's the charge nurse?" he asked, scowling. "Oh, there you are! The doctor told me this morning I was supposed to get some cough medicine. I haven't got it yet. Do you suppose I'm going to get it? Can you get it?"

"I'll check and see," the nurse said.

She went to the doctor's order book. Not understanding the order, she asked a few nurses about it and then inquired further about the use of the

Reprinted, with permission, from *The American Journal of Nursing*, LXIII, Aug. 1963, 56-59.

drug. After writing the drug card and ordering the medicine, she returned and told the patient his medication would arrive in a few minutes. About a half hour later it arrived, and the proper dosage was given to him.

"Thank you," he said with a smile. But had he really been helped? That is what I wanted to find out in this study.

I was not sure that patients' requests always clearly indicate their needs. If the patient is still in distress after the nurse assumed she has met his needs, and if she fails to ask questions about the meaning of the request or how her activity helped, the patient may not feel free to say he still needs help. Therefore, talking with patients after episodes like the one just described was part of my investigatory technique to find out whether patients really felt they had been helped by what was done for them.

When I asked this particular patient about how he felt, he replied:

"I need the cough medicine. I have had chronic sinusitis for 40 years. I have to irrigate my nose. All that mucus goes into my chest and I have to cough it up. I have to have a prostatectomy tomorrow, and I have to be able to breathe and cough and get the mucus up now, or I know the doctor won't do the operation. I've been waiting hours for the cough medicine. The doctor told me this morning at around 8:30 that he'd order it for me. Yes, I know what I need, that's why I asked the nurse. It's when I don't get the medicine that I get in trouble. I take care of it myself when I'm at home. I have all the equipment I need at home."

What had I found out?—that this patient knew what he needed to relieve his discomfort; that he could, therefore, clearly communicate a relevant request to the staff; that his irritation had stemmed from waiting to have the request fulfilled; and that he *had* been helped.

This study was carried out on adult medical and surgical wards of a large urban general hospital, where I observed 16 nurse-patient situations as they occurred. In each instance, after the nurse left the patient, I would ask him how he felt, whether or not he had been in distress, and whether the distress had been relieved by what the nurse had done, or still needed to be relieved.

This exploration involved several steps. First, I shared my observations with the patient to find out whether he was experiencing what I thought he was experiencing. If he admitted he was still in distress, I offered an activity I thought would relieve the distress. I then asked the patient whether or not he felt he had been helped.

As he talked, I continually watched for nonverbal as well as verbal clues. These nonverbal clues were most helpful; many patients seem to hesitate to be frank about what they think or how they feel. It was important not to *assume* any meaning, but to ascertain the meaning from the patient himself. Final observations that the patient looked better, as well as his saying that he felt better and why, were indications that the patient had been helped.

This process of exploration was adapted from the nursing process described by Ida Orlando in her book *The Dynamic Nurse-Patient Relationship*. Miss Orlando served as a consultant for this study.

The patient in the incident described above had been able to express his need and had been helped by the ensuing nursing activity. This did not, however, prove to be true with all the patients observed.

For instance, one patient told a nurse that he just couldn't sleep at night, and she said that she would get some sleeping medicine for him. He agreed to try it, but added that it really had never helped him. Ignoring his comment, she departed to obtain the medicine.

Then I asked the patient about his sleeping difficulty.

"I haven't slept for two nights," he said, suddenly pulling the bed sheet aside. "See, my heel is sore where it lies against the sheet. I just can't seem to get it in a position where it helps. It's always sore. For a couple days now it's been sore like this."

The patient had an injured knee and was lying on his back. He explained to me that he understood he must remain in this position.

I checked with the doctor and found that this patient could lie on his side and thus relieve the pressure on his heel. I explained this to the patient and helped him to a comfortable position on his side.

"This is so much better, Nurse," he exclaimed. "What a relief! Maybe I can sleep now. The pills never helped me."

He fell asleep within 20 minutes. Next day he said that he had not taken the sleeping medication, but had slept well for the first time in two days. He added that getting the pressure off his sore heel was what had helped.

This patient actually told the nurse that the sleeping medication had never helped, but the nurse left to get the medicine, anyway. Had she remained and asked more questions about the sleeping difficulty, she probably would have discovered the real problem and been able to help the patient.

Who knows why this patient couldn't express himself initially? Maybe he thought it was unreasonable to question the doctor since he thought the doctor wanted him to stay on his back. We don't really know. We only know that he needed help to express himself.

If the nurse caring for him had gone one step further to find out what the patient was really experiencing, she might have saved herself or other staff members added time and effort later on. For, if his need had not been met, it seems reasonable to assume that later he would have again called her or other staff members for this same problem.

Fourteen of the 16 patients included in the study admitted having been in distress. Five had initially expressed requests relevant to their distress and the latter had been relieved by the immediate nursing activity that had followed. The other nine patients, however, had not been able to express requests or comments clearly related to their distress until after I had explored the situation with them. Eight of these then stated that these explorations, or discussions, had helped them.

A ninth patient's distress could not be relieved because his need—dental service—could not be met as immediately as he would have liked. Nevertheless, after he and I had explored the situation, he indicated that he felt somewhat better after venting his feelings.

If he had not had an opportunity to express his anger, we might wonder if this unrelieved tension would have caused him to make more demands on the evening staff. We don't know. But we do know he felt better after discussing his feelings.

These findings seem to indicate that, even though basic nursing care may help patients, exploration to find out from a patient how he feels, what he thinks he needs, and whether he feels he has been helped is necessary in order to be sure that the patient is helped.

Faye Abdellah and Eugene Levine found that patients' complaints tend to be concentrated on familiar daily life, varying widely from the noise of TV and radio to the quality of the food (Hospitals 31, Nov. 1957.) They found that such complaints may not always suggest the kind of nursing care the patients need.

Similar findings are reported by Ernest Dichter, who adds that the complaints are a plaintive cry echoing fear and insecurity. (Mod. Hosp. 83, Sept. 1954.)

Esther Lucile Brown believes that the hospital must undergo drastic changes in its handling of patients in order to treat the man instead of the disease. (Newer Dimensions of Patient Care. Part I. The Use of the Physical and Social Environment of the General Hospital for Therapeutic Purposes, 1961.)

Nursing care should focus on patients as individuals, for these studies suggest that, even when it seems that the basic nursing care has been given, the patient may not be regarded as cured because he does not regard himself as cured. It is perhaps not surprising that we so often hear, "Nurse the patient, not his illness."

An analysis of the kinds of patient distresses revealed by this study showed that 13 of the 14 patients expressed adverse reactions to the hospital setting, while only one patient expressed feelings of distress stemming from the illness itself. When the patients were asked how long these distresses had been on their minds, their answers indicated a range of from 3 minutes to 9 days.

The time averaged about 11 hours in the group relieved by the basic nursing care, as compared with an average of about 40 hours in the group unrelieved by the basic nursing care.

Of the 13 patients who showed adverse reactions to the hospital setting, all were found to have either misunderstandings about the illnesses, treatments, diagnostic tests and procedures, or adverse reactions to a delay in nursing help or treatment. This raises the question of whether the very fact that the nurse carried out activities without attempting to secure information from the patient may have contributed to the development of these adverse reactions. If the nurse had tried to find out what the patient was experiencing, it seems that he might not have developed these misunderstandings or, if he had, that the misunderstandings might have been resolved.

The staff-patient ratios on the wards were determined for the time the data were being collected. The time consumed by the nurse-patient interactions and the investigator-patient interactions was also determined. An analysis of the data suggests that the effectiveness of the nursing activities was unrelated to the number of nursing personnel or to the length of time devoted to each patient. It appears, then, that it is not the length of time with the patient that determines effectiveness, but the method of nursing.

This conclusion is borne out by New, Nite, and Callahan, who found that patient attitudes about nursing care did not seem to vary with variations in the staff-patient ratio. (*Nursing Service and Patient Care: A Staffing Experiment*, 1959.) One reason offered for this was that there is an overemphasis on nursing functions, or that nurses are task-oriented rather than patient-oriented. Safford and Schlotfeldt report similar findings. Patients showed little change in their evaluation of nursing care under three different staffing patterns. (*Nurs. Res. 9,* Summer 1960.)

Exploration with a patient to ascertain his needs may take patience. "Why?" you may ask. Isn't it easy to find out what the patient is really thinking?

It is easy when patients know what they want and feel free to talk about it. But, if they are not clear about what they need, or if they think they should not question the care they are getting, then it becomes more difficult to find out what they need.

For example, the patient may be very quiet, and the nurse may feel that she is prying if she continues to question him. Or he may talk incessantly about seemingly irrelevant subjects, making the nurse feel he is repetitive or is taking her in circles. In such cases, the nurse may feel confused and leave. If she can say what she is thinking, she may be able to help the patient become clearer. For example, she might say, "I think we're going in circles. I don't understand exactly what you are trying to say," and then offer thoughts about what she thinks he might be trying to say.

The nurse's reactions and the patient's reactions will vary from situation to situation. No generalizations can be made. Each nurse may have to think about what is happening to her before she can get any ideas about how to help the patient.

How, then, can the nurse, who is often pressed by many duties, take the time to ask the patient the meaning of his request or comments? Is it worth the added time that might be involved? Let's look at one final example.

A patient was complaining of pain and pointed to her abdomen. The nurse remembered that the patient had recently had a cesarean section and assumed that the pain was from the incision. She nodded, said she'd get some medicine for the pain, and left the room.

In the meantime a student nurse entered the room. Again the patient said, "I have pain," and pointed to her abdomen. The student, who was not yet allowed to give medicine, moved closer to the bed and said, "Well, tell me where the pain is. Maybe there's something we can do about it."

The patient stammered. The student encouraged her to say what she was thinking.

Finally the patient blurted, "Well, you see, I hate to admit this, but I put on a three-way stretch girdle this morning, and I don't think the doctor will like it. You see, when I put it on I felt something funny happening." The patient squirmed. "I think my incision may have burst open. The doctor will be furious. I don't know what to do!"

"Let's look and see," said the student. With the student's help, the patient removed the girdle, and both could see that the stitches were all intact.

"Oh, I'm *so* relieved! The doctor would have been furious."

At this point the regular staff nurse returned with the medicine. The patient looked at the nurse and said, "Gee, I'm sorry, but the pain's gone now. I won't need that." She smiled.

This example shows that the nurse who had not found out what the patient was really thinking had taken time for an activity that would not have helped the patient. The student took a comparable length of time, found out what the patient was thinking, and met the patient's need. Had the need not been met, probably the patient would have called other staff members for help, taking even more nursing time. Any added time that might be initially taken in talking with the patient might save time in the long run.

The main point about this exploration is that the nurse shares her observations with the patient to find out whether he is experiencing what she thinks he is experiencing. If he hesitates at all, she might even say, "You're hesitating, I wonder if something more than what you've told me is on your mind." The main purpose is to clarify communication. Similar explorations can be carried on between instructors and students, with any medical personnel, or wherever there seems to be unclear communication.

The nurse dealing with a patient can ask herself after she leaves him:

What did I do and what did I say?

Why did I do these things, and why did I say these things?

What did I think they would accomplish?

What did they accomplish? In other words, how does this patient look now, compared to when I first saw him?

If he seemed to be in distress, does he look better?

If not, maybe I still have some questions to ask him about himself.

If the effectiveness of this exploration to find out what the patient is experiencing is confirmed by other studies, it may imply that nursing schools should allow time for their students to learn how to determine patients' immediate needs. Measuring the student's effectiveness in this activity could then be a further means of testing the student's nursing ability. For when we speak of "nursing effectiveness," we cannot omit the appraisal of the patient himself. It would seem that the aims of nursing are realized when a patient says, as one patient said to one nurse:

"I wasn't even sure what it was that I needed until you started talking with me and asking me these questions about how I looked and how I felt. You helped me to realize what was really bothering me. I feel so much better now!"

As examples of how nurses are trying to deal with patient problems, some approaches to specific groups of patients are presented. Papers 39 and 40 deal with children—one author using a psychoanalytic approach, the other using different theoretical avenues, including consideration of sensory deprivation. Paper 38 discusses problems in psychiatric nursing and paper 41 deals with nursing the aged. The last paper in this section is about the patient's concern with death.

38.
Interpersonal Techniques: The Crux of Psychiatric Nursing

by Hildegard E. Peplau

The time is past when a nurse could become, in one lifetime, an expert in all clinical areas. Advances in all fields of knowledge and within nursing science itself point to the inevitability of clinical specialization.

When you begin to think about specialization, however, you think not only of a focus in a particular area but of considerable depth. As the scope of the specialists' work narrows, the depth intensifies at, I submit, the point of the uniqueness of the clinical area. The unique aspect of a clinical area is twofold: it is that which occurs in other clinical fields but is not emphasized to the same extent and it is that which is almost entirely new—the uncommon, promising developments which result from thinking deeply about a particular facet of work in just one area.

Each of the areas of nursing practice has a particular clinical emphasis. This emphasis does not preclude attention to all the other aspects of the workrole of the nurse practitioner, but more time, effort, and thought are given to this particular facet. For example, nurses in public health programs emphasize health teaching, not to the exclusion of the technical aspects of nursing practice nor of the supportive, reassuring, mother-surrogate type of nurse activities. But, by and large, nurses who visit patients in their homes spend a proportionately larger part of their time teaching. Medical-surgical nursing emphasizes technical care; pediatric nursing emphasizes the mother-surrogate role; in this paper I want to consider the particular emphasis of psychiatric nursing.

I have indicated various subroles of the workrole of nurses. Briefly, these include mother-surrogate, technician, manager, socializing agent, health teacher, and counselor or psychotherapist.

Psychiatric nursing emphasizes the role of counselor or psychotherapist. It is true that this idea is not a universally accepted one in all psychiatric facilities. But note that I say "psychiatric nursing," not "nursing in psychiatric units."

There are two levels of professional nurse personnel practicing in psychiatric units—general practitioners (general duty nurses) and specialists (psychiatric nurses). Let me clarify the difference. A general practitioner is a nurse who has completed only her basic professional preparation. From my

Reprinted, with permission, from *The American Journal of Nursing*, LXII, June 1962, 50–54.

234

viewpoint, a "psychiatric nurse" is a specialist and at this time specialist status can be achieved by two routes—experience and education.

Before the passage of the Mental Health Act in 1946, experience was the route by which a nurse earned the title "psychiatric nurse"; since 1946, however, some 25 graduate-level, university-based programs in advanced psychiatric nursing have been established. There are stipends available for study in these programs. Any nurse who can qualify—because she has completed her full basic professional preparation and has the intellectual and personal qualifications for graduate study—can secure a stipend for graduate study toward becoming a clinical specialist in psychiatric nursing, that is, a "psychiatric nurse." From my point of view, then, the route of clinical specialization for any nurse who was graduated since 1946 is through a university-based graduate level program.

I realize this is a status problem but the profession of nursing will strengthen its position in relation to all other professional disciplines when it recognizes the culturally accepted fact that university education is the route for clinical specialization. There is good reason for this. Theoretically the university is free of the service commitment of the hospital—it can take objective distance, look dispassionately at the work of nurses, and dare to consider gross changes in the workrole.

When you are employed in a service agency, on the other hand, you become a participating member in its social system, ties of friendship and loyalty become binding as well as blinding, and dispassionate inquiry is greatly lessened. There is another reason why universities have culturally been charged with graduate education: the scope of established and newly formulated knowledge represented in a university faculty is ever so much wider than that represented in a professional staff group. It is access to this knowledge and its application to clinical observations that transform the student into an expert clinician.

There is clear distinction then between nursing in a psychiatric unit (what a general duty nurse does), and psychiatric nursing (what an expert clinical practitioner does). This distinction should be kept in the foreground for in this paper I will refer to nurses and nursing, when speaking of the common and basic elements, and to psychiatric nurses and psychiatric nursing when speaking of the more specialized clinical functions.

A psychiatric nurse is first of all an expert clinician. She may also be a teacher, supervisor, administrator, consultant, or researcher, but underlying all these functional positions there should be advanced clinical training. Such clinical expertness revolves around the field's unique aspect or emphasis, in this case, the role of counselor or psychotherapist. I want to develop the importance of this idea for the general practice of nursing in a psychiatric setting, but, first, I wish to pinpoint why other aspects of the work in a psychiatric unit are not the central focus of psychiatric nursing.

The emphasis in psychiatric nursing is *not* on the mother-surrogate role. Some nurses believe that the unmet needs of a patient's infancy and early childhood can be met by the nurse taking on various mothering activities. This belief assumes that the corrective experience is largely an emotional one resulting from a relationship in which the nurse complements a need for mothering of the patient, by supplying its counterpart—need-reducing mother-surrogate activities. This is analogous to the notion that when calcium deficiency produces tooth decay, supplying the calcium will fill up the cavities! A patient needs love, warmth, acceptance, support, and reassurance—not to supply the unmet needs of the past but for current reasons; having these emotional experiences makes it possible for the patient to come to grips with the earlier unmet needs on intellectual rather than on experiential grounds.

The notion that a made-up "good mother" experience will correct the patient's pathology is based on the assumption that the patient has not moved ahead in other areas compatible with chronological development—for example, language, vocabulary, and thought develop despite emotional deprivations.

To give mother-surrogate activities the central emphasis would be to de-emphasize these tools which have developed and can be utilized.

There is another inescapable fact; the small number of professional nurses in psychiatric facilities has for a long time required that the necessary mother-surrogate activities—the bathing, feeding, dressing, toileting, warning, disciplining, and approving the patient—be taken over largely by nonprofessional nursing personnel. I do not forsee that any great benefit would accrue even if the supply was such that professional nurses could take on fully these mothering activities. Note that I have not said that a nurse never bathes or feeds or dresses or warns a patient in a psychiatric unit; what I have said is that these mothering activities are not the central focus.

The emphasis in psychiatric nursing is *not* on the technical subrole. Some nurses believe that the cause of mental illness will ultimately prove to be some biochemical or otherwise organic problem, identifiable by the results of various laboratory test procedures and correctable by some technical manipulations analogous to the injection of insulin in the therapeutic management of a person diagnosed as diabetic. Other nurses in the past and present have believed that technical expertness in giving tubs, packs, coma insulin and care in the pre- and post-phases of electroconvulsive therapy or lobotomy would lead to solutions to mental illness. Technical expertness in giving medication or carrying out procedures associated with nursing is, in my opinion, not the desirable emphasis in psychiatric nursing.

The emphasis in psychiatric nursing is *not* on managerial activities. Historically, these have been aspects of custodial care with restraint, protection, cleanliness, and order the dominant themes. Many of the housekeeping activities associated with these themes have been shifted not only to nonprofessional personnel but to work details made up of working patients as well. The housekeeping activities have given way to a host of clerical and receptionist activities, which nurses have taken on, and which presumably have to do with the management of the patient's environment in the interest of his care. I submit that the time is near at hand when administrators will recognize that these clerical and receptionist activities can be performed far better and more cheaply by a high school graduate; that these are not "professional" activities but instead are largely busywork which keeps the nurse away from direct contact with patients.

The emphasis in psychiatric nursing is *not* on socializing-agent activities, such as playing cards and games with patients, taking walks and watching TV with them and the like. In some basic schools of nursing, students are taught that these actvities are central in the work of the nurse; I submit that the preparation of a nurse is not required for such activities; that the use of a nurse's social experience as an interesting diversionary activity in the patient's daily life is not the best use of the time of a professional nurse. Nonprofessional nursing personnel, volunteers, and visitors can do this game-playing just as well as a nurse can. The professional education of the nurse is wasted; it is not needed to perform these activities which most laymen learn some time during their "teens."

Group activities along these lines might better be planned and carried out by the recreational department or some department other than nursing service (or nursing education since students are largely "used" for this purpose). I have not said that a professional nurse *never* plays cards with patients; however, these activities are not the central emphasis in psychiatric nursing and at most should take a bare minimum of the day's time of a professional nurse.

The emphasis in psychiatric nursing is *not* on health teaching although this subrole, in the workrole of the nurse, is an important one which needs to be developed further. I have pointed out that this is an important part of the work of nurses in public health. But the patients in the case load of these nurses are more often immediately able to use information than are patients in the psychiatric setting. Even so, teaching psychiatric patients about diet, nutrition, grooming, sex, and the like, may be very helpful. There has also been one promising study reported in which psychiatric patients were taught a concept of anxiety to apply to their own experiences; several similar studies are now under way.*

The emphasis in psychiatric nursing is on the counseling or psychotherapeutic subrole. This generalization is based upon the assumption that the difficulties in living which lead up to mental illness in a particular patient are subject to investigation and control by the patient—with professional counseling assistance. It is also based on a second assumption: that formal knowledge of counseling procedure is absolutely essential for the more general type of approach which may be useful in very brief relationships with patients. Further, these general approaches are in the nature of "interpersonal techniques" useful in relation to specific problems—such as withdrawal, aggression, hallucinations, delusions, and the like—and these are the crux of psychiatric nursing.

There is being developed in psychiatric nursing a theory and procedure of nurse counseling. This development is proceeding along two lines:

1. A "surface type" of formal counseling procedure, such as a general nurse practitioner might use with patients in all clinical areas, is being described. Many schools of nursing already are beginning to teach interviewing—of a therapeutic in contrast to a biographical type—as a basis for counseling. A companion result of this development will surely be the identification and description of a variety of general approaches to specific problems—interpersonal techniques—which nurses can use in everyday brief contacts with all types of patients.

2. Depth counseling, such as might be employed by a psychiatric nurse specialist who had completed two years of master's level clinical training, is also being described. Several nurses are now employed in situations in which they are doing long-term counseling of patients, utilizing the competencies secured through such clinical training. It is conceivable that in another decade or two nurses will share offices with psychiatrists and psychologists and social workers for the private practice of psychiatric nurse counseling, although now there are no publishable instances of such practices.

In many basic schools of nursing, students are being taught counseling technique in connection with nurse-patient care studies, particularly in the psychiatric setting. I have talked with a number of teachers in these schools and their general conclusion seems to be that when the student has an opportunity to work directly with one patient—say in one-hour sessions twice a week over a period of ten weeks—a great deal of learning takes place.

The student gets more than a textbook picture of pathology; she gets a full view of the complexity of the difficulties of a psychiatric patient, of the varia-

* See "Teaching a Concept of Anxiety," by Dorothea Hays in *Nursing Research*, Vol. 10, pp. 108-113, Spring 1961 issue.

tions which occur in particular patterns of behavior. Many students find out, for example, that there are infinite variations of the pattern of withdrawal and that observed changes in the behavior of a patient are more likely to be changes from one variant to another of a central pattern that persists. Thus, a patient who uses gross withdrawal—by muteness, for example—can, as a result of a nurse-patient relationship, eventually, begin to speak; the verbalizations, however, are also classifiable as a variant of withdrawal, particularly when the patient talks but doesn't communicate anything descriptive of his difficulties.

In a carefully guided nurse-patient relationship, the nurse learns the art and science of counseling technique. She discovers that the art part of it is intuitively based—it is a clinical judgment which she herself makes, minute by minute, that this maneuver or that maneuver might conceivably be useful to the investigative effort. The student also learns the value of knowledge and procedures for their application to explain observations; this is the scientific part. The student gradually ceases to use such terms as anxiety, conflict, dissociation, and the like, as mere labels for behavior; she begins to use these concepts as scientific tools to guide her in assessing the investigative effort under way and in getting more information. Both the nurse and patient need as much descriptive information about the patient's life experiences as can be obtained without making the patient too uncomfortable. It is this information which will be worked over by the nurse and patient together so that the patient can understand and benefit from his previous experiences in living.

Another important learning accrues from teaching counseling in the nurse-patient relationship. The student learns detachment; she learns—with the help of her teachers—how not to usurp the counseling time to meet her own needs; how to use the time instead, to help the patient formulate and meet his needs. She learns to make clearer distinction between techniques that are useful to her socially, outside the professional work situation, and those specifically useful in a clinical situation.

Moreover, the student learns a lot about herself as she begins to understand her reactions to the patients' behavior and verbal content, her own need for approval, the points at which she is particularly vulnerable. Patients have a way of unwittingly locating the vulnerabilities of students—be it their need for approval, their sensitivity to their appearance, their embarrassment in discussion about sex, or any one of a host of similar problem areas.

Once a student nurse has had successive counseling interviews with a particular patient, and has responsibly reviewed her nurse-patient data with an expert psychiatric nurse teacher, she is able to transfer—or generalize—the learning products to much briefer relationships with patients. Students invariably report that learning about counseling of one patient helps them to use to better advantage the two-to-three-minute contacts they have with patients in the ward setting. Nor do I know of any other way for a student to achieve these understandings except as a result of talking with one patient about the patient's difficulties, in designated, time-limited sessions occurring over a period of time, and following each session by a substantial review of what went on with an expert psychiatric nurse. You can't tell students what to do along these lines and then expect them, magically, to be able to do it. The student must not only experience this day-to-day process but she must have interested and active help in examining, bit by bit, the interview data which she thus collects.

One result, then, of the nurse-patient inquiry is the ability to transfer a substantial amount of learning toward more generalized interpersonal techniques. I believe that such techniques are the crux of psychiatric nursing and it seems to me that it ought to be possible for psychiatric nurses to develop specific interpersonal techniques useful in intervening in specific patterns of pathological behavior of patients. And it is possible; several nurses I know are currently involved in developing and testing such techniques.

One of the major difficulties of most, if not all, psychiatric patients is anxiety. We need a simple interpersonal technique which would be of value in the productive abatement of severe anxiety in patients. What might the steps of such a technique be? Could these steps be carried out by nonprofessional nursing personnel under the supervision of professional nurses who would have a deeper insight into the merits of the technique based upon the emotional experience of the nurse-patient investigation?

The steps are simple:

1. Encourage the patient to identify the anxiety as such. This is done by having all personnel help him recognize what he is experiencing at the point when he is actually anxious. Such anxiety is observable. In other words, the patient may well be unaware of his anxiety but another person—particularly a trained professional person—can observe the effects of anxiety and therefore infer its presence. So, a professional nurse would determine that a particular patient was anxious and unaware of it. Her behavior toward the patient and her supervision of the relationships which nonprofessional personnel have with him would be guided by the aim: to help the patient identify the anxiety as such. This would be done by saying to the patient, for as long as it takes to achieve the recognition, "Are you uncomfortable," "Are you nervous," "Are you upset," "Are you anxious?" With most psychiatric patients, it may take an amazingly long time to get a "Yes" answer, that is, to get him to recognize his anxiety. In many instances, the patient's responses will follow a sequence, beginning with "No" to "Sometimes I am," "Maybe," "A little," and finally,

"Yes, I am uncomfortable (or anxious)." When such "Yes" responses are obtained, the nurse can assume a modicum of awareness of anxiety; then, and not before then, the patient is ready for the second step in the interpersonal technique for utilizing anxiety constructively.

2. Encourage the patient to connect the relief-giving patterns that he uses to the anxiety which requires such relief. The nursing personnel focus their efforts on maintaining the patient's awareness of the anxiety and connecting it to his anxiety-relieving behavior. Thus, the nurse might observe that a patient was anxious. The nurse would ask, "Are you uncomfortable now?" If the patient replied, "Yes," the nurse would ask, "What do you do to get comfortable again when you are anxious?" This step would be repeated until it was clear to the professional observer that the patient did, indeed, formulate the connection between his anxiety and the anxiety-relieving behavior he uses. Describing this behavior, he might say, "I cry," "I swing my foot," "I pace," "I talk to voices," "I worry about my family," and the like.

Working in this manner with a particular patient, one graduate nurse student had the experience of hearing a patient say, "Yes, I am anxious right now, I am very anxious, I feel terrible, and I'm going over there and rock myself on that rocking chair good and hard and then I'll come back." A bit later, the patient did return to the nurse and commented, "Now I'm not so anxious; that rocking chair sure helps but I need to find out why I am anxious."

3. Encourage the patient to provide himself and the nurse with data descriptive of situations and interactions which go on immediately before an increase in anxiety is noticed. Once he has connected his anxiety-relieving behavior with his anxiety, the patient is ready for this third step: beginning the search for precipitating causes of the anxiety. Here the nursing personnel might ask, "What went on just before you got so uncomfortable?" The aim is to get the patient to describe the situations or interactions in which he was involved immediately preceding the developing increase in anxiety. Such description provides the nurse with a range of data about the patient so that she can begin to speculate (for herself) on probable causes of the anxiety.

Here, the application of the concept of anxiety—which defines areas of causation—would be useful for the professional nurse. It cannot be over emphasized that in this step the patient is not searching for immediate, situational causes of the increase in his anxiety; he is merely providing a description of experience from which such causes can later be inferred.

4. Encourage the patient to formulate from the descriptive data the probable immediate, situational causes for the increase in his anxiety.

In Step 3 the professional nurse can begin to speculate as to causes; helping the patient to formulate his own view of the reasons for his anxiety is

Step 4. Step 4 makes use of the descriptions which have accumulated out of several days of talks between the patient and the nursing personnel. The professional nurse might ask such questions as, "What have you noticed going on before you get anxious that might increase your discomfort?" Questions of this type encourage the patient to notice and to formulate cause-effect relations on his own.

Any patient who is able to utilize these four steps will show improvement in his ability to cope not only with living in the ward setting but with his pathology as well. Such a patient is most likely ready for a fifth step—referral for intensive counseling so that the causes of anxiety involving the connections between remote past experience and immediate situational experiences can be identified.

It is my premise that interpersonal techniques—such as the one I have indicated here—can be devised and utilized by nursing personnel in relation to problematic behavior patterns of psychiatric patients. I believe that these interpersonal techniques, rather than modifications of medical-surgical nursing techniques, are the crux of the practice of nursing in a psychiatric setting.

39.
Ego Support for the Child Patient

by Margo Smith

If you have ever given nursing care to a young, hospitalized child, no doubt you have wondered, "What can I do that will help him withstand all that is happening to him?" Many times we are giving more emotional support than we realize. Yet, at other times, because we underestimate what is happening, we omit an important element of emotional support.

Some theories and principles concerning the development of the child's personality have certain implications for the nurse's role in giving emotional support. By identifying some of the implications of this knowledge we can relate them in tangible ways to the effective emotional support the nurse gives the young hospitalized child.

Personality Development

Several concepts of personality structure as discussed by A. P. Noyes, may be used in examining the dynamics of how the personality functions. For

Reprinted, with permission, from *The American Journal of Nursing*, LXIII, October 1963, 90–95.

the purposes of this article we are following the concept proposed by Freud, who divided personality into id, ego, and super-ego. While Noyes makes it clear that the age at which personality appears is difficult to determine, some generalizations can be made about the personality components in the young child.

For the first two years of life, the child's personality is largely dominated by feelings and primitive instincts. This is the id portion of the personality. The young child demands immediate satisfaction of his desires and operates according to the pleasure principle. As the child becomes conscious of his own identity and of the demands of reality, the ego portion of the personality emerges and establishes a relationship with the world outside. The goals of the ego may be defined as: stabilizing between the instinctual drives and the demands of reality, and stabilizing between the instinctual drives and the socializing forces.

With respect to the development of the ego, Noyes points out the significance of the relationship between mother and child. It may even be postulated that, during the child's toddlerhood, the mother acts as his ego until he has acquired controls from within. This conscious, reasoning part of the personality becomes stronger as the personality matures, but may be weakened by fatigue, illness, and the strain of continued repression. Readily apparent is the fact that the undeveloped ego of the child, further weakened by illness and hospitalization, can hardly be expected to cope with unusual events in a realistic fashion without purposeful assistance.

The third hypothetical segment of the personality, the superego, is well advanced by the time the child is five. The superego, described as "the internalized agent of socializing forces," has the goal of criticizing the ego's acceptance of instinctual drives from the id. This is accomplished through authority figures, especially the child's family, and the child's responses to them become incorporated into his personality. *(Modern Clinical Psychiatry.* 4th ed., 1953.).

Within this framework we will attempt to identify the nurse's goal in giving emotional support to the young child. The amount and kind of emotional support the child will need, it seems, will depend on the strength of his ego; for his ego determines the way in which he will respond to internal and external forces.

Ego Support as the Goal

Ego support as used here denotes those nursing activities which assist the patient to cope with the demands of reality. It seems to be a definitive term and one that immediately calls to mind the purpose of emotional support—to assist the individual to maintain a reality orientation through his ability to perceive reality and to respond to it in his own way within his own limitations.

The two essential elements in providing ego support seem to be:

Allowing the child to be dependent. The infant's dependency on someone else is obvious; he is physically unable to meet his own needs and he is emotionally unable to tolerate having his needs unmet, even for a short period of time. Having his dependency needs met enables him to develop a sense of trust in his environment and, eventually, to develop a feeling of mastery over stressful situations. These feelings of trust and mastery contribute to the growth of his ego so that he can cope with reality situations, such as waiting a while for his feeding.

Dependency is not forced upon him; rather, he is allowed to be dependent until he can develop the strengths necessary to be independent and interdependent. Even as he grows older, having his dependency needs met serves to help the child acquire feelings of trust and mastery about a situation. Much stress, however, must be placed on merely allowing, rather than imposing, dependency. Dependency on someone involves feelings of helplessness, so that an effort is made to meet dependency needs without making the child feel totally helpless. Allowing the child to be dependent appears to be one of the first steps in supporting his ability to cope with reality, or in supporting his ego.

Assisting the child to develop independency. At certain ages the child becomes ready to learn certain things. A built-in desire to learn and to achieve makes some of the child's learning experiences thoroughly enjoyable for him. However, when he must forfeit pleasure for the purpose of meeting the demands of reality, he naturally experiences a degree of frustration. If he is physically and psychologically ready to manage the frustration of the new learning situation, then the experience will provide him with another mastery over his environment and equip him with more ego resources with which to meet the demands of reality.

Implications of Ego Support

There are certain areas in the child's life during a hospital experience in which the implications of ego support can be used to help him.

Maintaining a relationship with his mother. Because of hospital rules or inconvenience to the family, the child's hospitalization often means separation from the family. Yet, the stress of illness and hospitalization places a premium on continuing a close relationship between parent and child; for, as we have seen, the child's beginning ability to cope with reality situations is fashioned within the parent-child relationship.

Bowlby describes the effects of a child being deprived of a warm and continuous relationship with his mother. Even partial deprivation brings acute anxiety, excessive need for love, and feelings of revenge and guilt, all of which are evidence of psychic disorganization. Studies reported by Bowlby *(Maternal Care and Mental Health,* 1951) clearly indicate that, although vulnerability to maternal deprivation slowly diminishes with age, at least by the time the child has reached six months of age and until he is five years old, he is seriously vulnerable to the effects of maternal deprivation.

An hypothesis of an ego-supporting nursing activity is that the nurse encourages a continuous parent-child relationship and remains alert to the adverse effects of deprivation. The nurse works closely with the mother, encouraging her to visit often and informing her of whatever visiting restrictions exist in the hospital. Of utmost importance to the child and his family is the nurse's planning with the family in regard to who will be able to visit the child and when the visit is to take place. The child needs to be visited by both parents together, for seeing their relationship is a most supporting thing to him. The family unit is the young child's primary environment, molding his ability to cope with reality. The nurse needs to know when the parent is returning so that she can, periodically, as the need arises, graphically explain to the young child when he can expect his parent again. The young child is often fearful that the parent will not return, and many fear that hospitalization is a punishment inflicted by the parents.

The Use of Purposeful Play

Play for children has long been of undisputed value. Virtually every book on childhood growth and development emphasizes the educational and emotional importance of play. Equally important also is that play is probably the most independent activity in which a young child can engage. It is one of the few things a young child does which involves only minimal interference by the adult. It is not surprising then that play for the ill and hospitalized child can be a beneficial tool in assisting the child to adjust to the stressful situation.

E. H. Erickson states that "to play it out is the most natural, self-healing measure childhood affords." *(Childhood Society,* 1950.) Piaget explains that play which repeats painful states is for the purpose of rendering pain "bearable, even pleasurable, through assimilation to the whole activity of the ego." *(Play, Dreams and Imitations in Childhood,* 1952.) Barton examines the hypothesis "that situational doll play can reduce the anxiety-producing effects of hospital experiences in children." *(Nursing Outlook 10,* March 1962.) Such statements as these have implications for nursing activities.

An hypothesis of an ego-supporting nursing activity might be that the nurse provides the child with an opportunity to play with and examine the equipment and procedures involved in his hospital experience. Such types of play may not visibly affect his response to the stressful situations, but there is reason to believe that the play experience will relieve him of some tension and will assist him to assimilate reality.

Further support of the child's need to become reality-oriented is Anna Freud's statement that the small child reacts more to fantasy aroused by the procedure than to the procedure itself. *(In Psychoanalytic Study of the Child,* 1952.) The child may have considerably inaccurate fantasies about both the stressful situation itself and the purpose of it. Many examples of this are discussed in an article by Florence Erickson. She found, for instance, that the pre-school child perceived the adult administering rectal and parenteral procedures as being hostile in intent, not protective. *(Nursing Outlook 6,* Sept. 1958.)

Another possible hypothesis of an ego-supporting nursing activity in relation to play is that the nurse provides play involving toys from home and stories which remind the child of pleasant home experiences. Encouraging the family to bring toys from home not only assists the family to feel that they can help the child, but also provides the child with a source of emotional comfort. Certainly, the familiar, ragged, cuddly doll from home is far more valuable to the child than any type of doll the hospital could provide.

The Child's Learning Activities

The fact that the young child has dependency-independency conflicts is well known to all who have studied growth and development. This factor in the normal child is further complicated in the ill and hospitalized child who experiences additional anxiety. Adler explains that anxiety precipitates a striving for both dependence and independence. *(Understanding Human Nature,* 1927.)

An hypothesis of an ego-supporting nursing activity is that the nurse assists the child in continuing previously learned activities and in learning further about the reality situation of illness and hospitalization. The child experiences feelings of pride, independence, and power in connection with many of the things he has learned to do for himself. Whenever possible the time should be taken to allow the child to continue to do these things for himself. Several factors, however, influence this situation. Certainly there will be times when the child needs to be dependent and when he will indicate that he wants the nurse to do things for him that he has already learned to do for himself.

Hospitalization and illness present many new things for the child to learn and we have seen that these may be complicated by a great deal of fantasy.

the child to stop crying or stop pouting only conveys to the child that he is not understood and that he will receive no help with his feelings.

The child's aggressive behavior in response to frustration may also be dealt with by the nurse verbalizing that she understands the behavior which may consist of kicking or hitting. When the child demonstrates behavior that cannot be tolerated in view of the nurse's safety or the child's safety, the nurse helps the child substitute appropriate channels for the outlet of aggressive behavior, such as kicking a ball or a doll.

Distracting the child during stressful periods has its place, but the nurse must use skilled judgment. During a period of acute anxiety, the child is consumed with what is happening to him. The immediate situation concerns him most, and the nurse's most appropriate response may be to talk to him about what occupies his attention at this time. For example, during a painful experience, the nurse can tell the child what is happening and how soon it will be over. When it is over, the child needs to be told that it is over, for he may continue to fear that the pain will recur. Then distraction is needed, but only when the child's anxiety is not acute. The nurse attempts to distract the child only when his mind can truly be directed at another subject.

The presence of the nurse, in itself, may meet one of the child's needs during a period of anxiety. Schachter says that the desire to be with another person increases as anxiety increases. *(The Psychology of Affiliation,* 1959.)

The purposeful use of touch, such as cuddling the child or holding his hand, can be an effective means of meeting the child's dependency needs and of showing him love and affection. Fenichel says that for some persons, the warmth of physical contact or touch is a means of receiving affection. He further states that foregoing the pleasure of touch is the ego's way of learning to master reality. *(The Psychoanalytic Theory of Neurosis,* 1945.) During periods of stress the child may benefit from touch due to his need to be dependent. The use of touch, however, must be understood and be purposeful; for a child who resists touch has an equally important need to be independent.

Meeting Physical Needs

The importance of meeting physical needs in infancy is readily seen. The importance of this aspect of care applies not only to the age of almost complete dependency but also to situations encountered throughout life when the child or adult must depend on someone else to meet his physical needs.

Another hypothesis of an ego-supporting nursing activity is that the nurse meets the physical needs of the child promptly so that he will have energy available for coping with other anxiety and consequently be able to utilize his energy for the purpose of getting well. This hypothesis incorporates the basis for being able to perform all other ego-supporting nursing activities.

Learning is possible, however, and can be beneficial. Towle explains that learning is a positive and innate tendency and serves to ease anxiety and to contribute to feelings of self-sufficiency and safety. (*Common Human Needs,* 2d ed., 1952.) Providing opportunities for the young child to participate in procedures is one means of assisting him to learn, to cope with reality, and to feel a measure of independence. Even the toddler can feel that he is participating in a procedure when he is provided with an opportunity to do such things as hold a basin for an irrigation or hold a gauze flat during a dressing change.

In addition to the use of play and participation, the nurse helps the child cope with and learn about reality simply by giving him appropriate choices, by being honest with him, and by utilizing a positive approach. For example, when the child is to undergo a painful procedure, the nurse tells him that it will be uncomfortable, or uses some other appropriate word, such as sting, and tells him gently, but positively, that it will be done. The young child cannot be asked if he is ready for the painful procedure or if he wants it done. Such questions would impose too much responsibility on the young child, besides implying a choice when there is none.

Honest explanations help the child learn about reality, therefore, contributing somewhat to a lessened anxiety and a degree of safety and independence. An honest approach about pain will undoubtedly upset the child at the time; however, it has a far-reaching effect upon the child's trust and confidence in the nurse.

Going ahead with the procedure as soon as possible reduces the amount of anxiety and frustration the child experiences, especially if he perceives the procedure as painful or assaulting. Studies show that as the time approaches for the subject to engage in a stressful activity, feelings of anxiety increase. The child's limited time perception also contributes to the need to perform the procedure as soon as possible.

The Child's Natural Responses

Regardless of what causes anxiety to the child, his natural reaction will be to strike out at the frustration and to avoid it. An hypothesis of an ego-supporting nursing activity is that the nurse accepts the child's behavior in response to frustration as being natural and that the nurse responds to the child's dependency-independency conflict.

In order to accept the child's behavior in response to frustration as being natural, the nurse must first be convinced herself that such behavior is indeed natural. The nurse is then able to tell the child that she knows the situation hurts or bothers him and that all children respond with anger or fear. Telling

Maslow outlines a hierarchy of basic human needs and describes physiological needs as undoubtedly the most prepotent of all needs. They must be at least partially met before other needs emerge, such as safety needs, love needs, and esteem needs. *(Psychol. Rev. 50,* July 1943.). Many physiological needs involve direct physical care and touch. If these needs are met promptly and in such a way that the child feels loved, the activity becomes ego-supporting and the child feels mastery over reality.

40.

The Meaning of Maternal Deprivation and Separation Anxiety for Nursing Practice

by Dorothy Johnson

Maternal deprivation and separation anxiety are still rather nebulous concepts in some respects, despite numerous studies to be found in the literature. Most of these studies are on a descriptive level and have provided substantial evidence that deprivation of maternal care, including a break in the continuity of the mother-child relationship, particularly in the first 36 months of life, not only may result in immediate behavioral reactions but may have permanent aftereffects. We have little basis, at this point, for questioning either the existence or the importance of this general phenomenon. Deriving effective nursing practices from this knowledge is a tenuous matter, however, for as yet we have very little knowledge of the basic processes involved in this relationship. Although we have some notion of what the problem is, we know very little of why, or how, or even when. Practice based on "what" can be gained only through trial and error, while practice based on "why" and "how" offers greater promise of effectiveness. Ongoing research in at least two seemingly unrelated areas offers hope in this regard. I believe these investigations, among others, have very real potential for clarifying the essential nature of the mother-child relationship and its underlying mechanisms.

Harlow, at Wisconsin, has undertaken to explore experimentally the nature of love, in terms of the development of affectional responses by infant monkeys to an artificial mother. Perhaps the most important of his findings reported to date, a finding which may have relevance to man, is the great

From a paper read at the 1962 clinical sessions of the American Nurses' Association and published in monograph No. 2, *Nursing in Relation to the Impact of Illness on the Family.* ANA, 1962, 23–33.

importance of body contact with a soft, warm, figure as an affectional variable. He has found, for example, that infant monkeys spend considerable time in contact with their terry-cloth-covered mother surrogates even if they have to leave her for feeding from a wire mother. Contact, to Harlow, seems to have greater value than nursing in the development of an affectional tie between the infant monkey and his mother. Further, in the face of fear-arousing stimuli, contact with the cloth mother provides sufficient comfort to the infant monkey to enable him to explore the fearful object or situation visually and even manipulatively. The wire mother, even a wire mother that feeds, does not provide the same kind of security; indeed, in the same fear-producing situation with only the wire mother on hand, the infant monkey retreats into himself, rocking, clutching himself, and vocalizing. Jean M. Arsenian found in her work with nursery children aged 11-30 months that they responded to a strange room in much the same way; when they were alone, the children spent the time in crying or in autistic behavior; in the presence of their mothers, the children displayed behavior evaluated as symptomatic of security. (*Journal of Abnormal and Social Psychology 38,* April 1943.) Harlow is continuing his work with respect to other affectional variables, including clinging, rocking, and the effects of consistency and inconsistency with the mother-surrogate. His research should do much to elucidate the bases of affection and the mechanisms underlying affectional ties.

The second area in which much interesting work is going on is variously referred to as sensory deprivation, perceptual isolation, and social isolation. In brief, this research—stimulated in part by recent developments in space technology—is concerned with the effects of reduced or patterned sensory stimulation on perceptual, cognitive, and psycho-social functioning. The findings are indeed striking, although conclusions are not yet possible. When the sensory input of healthy adults is reduced or strongly patterned by such means as solitary confinement in a dark room or restriction of movement in a respirator, they are unable in many instances to maintain their normal patterns of functioning beyond a few hours. They show emotional disturbances with delusions and mental imagery, there are gross distortions in perception, and significant impairment in cognitive functioning. While their "recovery" is usually rather rapid on return to the "normal" environment, the research raises many questions relative to the importance of sensory stimulation, including that inherent in social interaction, in the maintenance of function—physiologically, psychologically, and socially. That this work bears a strong relationship to the phenomenon of maternal deprivation was suggested long before our recent active interest in "man in space." Harry Bakwin suggested in 1942 (*American Journal of Diseases of Children 63,* Jan. 1942), and again in 1949 (*Journal of Pediatrics 35,* Oct. 1949), that infants' failure to thrive in institutions, including hospitals, might well be due to a general lack of stimulation, and he sites Chapin, Parrot, and Czerny as early proponents of this notion.

It is highly likely that the global term "maternal deprivation" may be reduced to a number of more discrete components by research such as this. This is important not only because the phenomenon thus becomes more amenable to research, but also because the findings may then provide us with a sounder basis for nursing intervention. There is, for example, the suggested importance of body contact; perhaps, a particular kind of sensory stimulation of the skin is essential to physiological functioning as well as to the development of affectional ties and psychological functioning. There is also the possibility of greater understanding of the importance of variety in sensory stimuli for proper functioning of the central nervous system and for the development and continuous correction of the perceptual and conceptual models on which we depend in coping with the world in which we live.

A description of maternal deprivation and its effects is relatively easy to provide because of the vast literature available. It is apparently a relative rather than an absolute condition in most instances, associated with neglect or rejection as well as physical separation. John Bowlby defines maternal deprivation as a state of affairs in which the child does not have "a warm, intimate, and continuous relationship with his mother (or permanent mother substitute) in which both find satisfaction and enjoyment." *(Maternal Care and Mental Health,* Monograph Series No. 2, 1951.) He amplifies this by reference to a deprivation of mother love. The physical care that the child receives may be adequate in the sense that such basic needs as those for food, warmth, and protection from injury or infection are met. It is interesting to note in this regard a common theory among behavioral scientists: the underlying mechanism of the infant's attachment to his mother is that of learning based on primary drive reduction. Both Harlow's work and reports of a number of clinical observers that some infants fail to thrive with adequate physical care would seem to negate this theory.

A cluster of immediate behavioral reactions, when separation of mother and child occurs, has been delineated particularly for the 6-to-36 month age group, and the term separation anxiety has been used to refer to this syndrome. H. R. Schaffer, *(British Journal of Medical Psychology 31, 1958),* however, describes two different syndromes, dependent on age: 1) the global syndrome which occurs in infants under seven months; and 2) the over-dependent syndrome in infants over seven months. He believes the first syndrome is related to perceptual deprivation and only the second is related to maternal deprivation. While Bowlby and others point to differences dependent on age, he tends to classify all reactions in three time-sequence stages: protest, despair, and denial. With some minor variations, the observations of other investigators seem to follow this pattern.

In the initial period of protest, the child tends to cry vigorously and his crying may or may not decrease on contact with an adult. He is likely to call for his mother loudly and repeatedly and to react negatively to other adults. In a day or two, the intermediate stage of despair begins in which the child tends to cry less, and there may be long intervals of quiet and subdued behavior. Some evidence of regressive behavior may be observed and there may be loss of appetite and weight. The child may continue to ignore the adults around him or he may make ceaseless demands for contact but without emotional response. He will cling to any tangible evidence of home—a doll, a blanket, or mother's hankie. It is also in this stage that intercurrent infection is likely to occur. The last stage of detachment is characterized by an increasing delay in response to the mother when she visits; the seeking of positive relationships with others, often on a rather superficial level; an increased interest in the sweets or toys his mother brings; and an increase in autoerotic behavior. Rene Spitz (see his articles in *Psychoanalytic Study of the Child,* vols. 1 and 2), and L. K. Fischer (*American Journal of Orthopsychiatry 22,* July 1952), have found, in addition, a serious gradual decline in the developmental quotient during these stages.

While some children go through a separation experience apparently unscathed and unaffected, many not only demonstrate the behavior described above during the separation, but also manifest continuing disturbance after reunion with the mother. These mild-to-moderate effects, which last from a few days to several months, take the form of somatic disturbances and alterations in eating and sleeping patterns, excessive clinging to the mother and demands for attention, fear of strangers and the like. In instances where the effects are severe, object relations are disturbed; reality testing is grossly disturbed; primary process thinking is prominent; and the drive-ego balance is unfavorable. These children appear emotionally withdrawn and isolated; they have few ties or friendships; they are social only in a superficial sense. Their behavior is impulsive; their capacity for inhibition and for abstract thinking is impaired; and they are unable to learn from experience. This damage to the developing organism may be irreversible. In the very young child, death may follow severe or prolonged deprivation.

A number of factors seem to influence the reaction to and effects of maternal deprivation. Of these, age has received the greatest attention and it seems reasonably certain that the first 36 months of life are of crucial importance. Other factors perhaps are significant though less is known about them and findings to date are not as unequivocal. We might mention the length of separation and its character, i.e., whether it is complete or partial. The pre-separation mother-child relationship and child-adaptive capacity, the parental attitude toward and reaction to the separation, and parental management of the child following the separation, have all been suggested as important. The separation environment and the child's management by the responsible adults in that environment also have been considered, and these factors are of vital interest to us. And, of course, we cannot forget the stresses associated with the illness itself.

Now, what does all this mean for nursing practice? Are these findings which we can utilize in the management of this problem? Some of the changes made in hospital policies in recent years have been based, at least in part, on this knowledge and on some associated assumptions. Visiting hours for parents have been liberalized and facilities for "rooming-in" have been provided. Professionally directed play programs have been developed. Planned programs of preparation for admission for children and their parents have been instituted. Staff personnel have been encouraged, in a general sense, to respond to the "emotional needs" as well as the physical and medical needs of the child. Unfortunately, the effects of these newer practices have not been, and perhaps can not all be, studied systematically to any extent with respect to the phenomenon of maternal deprivation; they are rather general in nature and pose problems for measurement. Nonetheless, these are important changes in the direction of better care for children in hospitals, even though not all of them may have direct bearing on our problem.

There are other quite concrete and specific nursing practices which might be initiated and studied, however. At this time, these must be based as much on hunch as on knowledge but there is some reason to believe they may hold promise. Let me cite several examples: Linda had been hospitalized, with the exception of a two-week period shortly after birth, for her entire four months. She had multiple congenital anomalies, the most immediately urgent of which were the genitourinary tract and would require corrective surgery. She had had repeated bouts of infection. At four months she seemed completely apathetic. She did not respond to either the people or the objects in her environment. She lay motionless in her bed unless moved. She ate but showed no interest in either the food or the feeder. She weighed only seven pounds. Her physical care had been quite adequate, and her medical needs had been met with conscientiousness and dispatch. Linda could not be called an attractive or appealing baby, and her prognosis was exceedingly poor. The parents, who were quite young, had one other child, 10 months older than Linda. They were aware of Linda's prognosis and seemed to have gradually cut their ties to her for they visited less and less frequently until they did not come at all. The nursing staff also seemed to have cut their ties to Linda as an individual being. Her care shifted from one to another from day to day and she was given little attention beyond that required to meet her physical or medical needs. The staff's collective attitude was one of hopelessness; they were literally unable to see how anything could possibly make a difference; and besides, they were "really quite busy." They were agreeable, however, to the proposal that a volunteer spend some time with Linda.

A warm and motherly older woman, a volunteer who had previously given much of her free time to work with us on the pediatric unit, agreed to help us with Linda. She began to visit the infant several times a day and tried to be on hand for her feedings; she even came on weekends whenever possible. Each visit was not very long but she fed Linda, cuddled and rocked her, and sang her songs. She frequently changed the position of Linda's bed and carried her to the window, around the room, and down the corridor. Sometimes she just sat holding Linda and talking to her softly, and the baby often went to sleep in her arms. In about three weeks Linda was a markedly changed baby. She was following people and objects with her eyes, smiling in response to overtures from others, lifting and turning her head, and attempting to move her body. She had gained in weight and continued to gain slowly. In another few weeks, Linda was so much better physically that the surgeons decided to go ahead and operate. Linda did not survive this experience but what had happened to her made a tremendous impact on all of us.

Debbie offered a different picture and a different problem. She was admitted at age two because of severe malnutrition. The quality of her previous maternal care was open to question, both within her own home and the other homes in which she had been placed for short periods from time to time. She came from a family of several children and very low income, one that was "on the move" almost constantly. Her parents had undoubtedly done the best they could for Debbie but they were too caught up in their own problems, both personal and economic, to provide the care she needed. Despite her scrawny appearance and the withdrawn quality of her interactions, several members of the nursing staff were drawn at once to Debbie. She blossomed with the constant attention and tender care she received. This was not the usual care given to all children; it had some special qualities and characteristics. There were frequent contacts with a few people who remained pretty constant in Debbie's orbit. Their interactions exuded warm interest and personal involvement. They provided Debbie with a variety of obviously satisfying social experiences and new opportunities. These nurses played with Debbie, in her room, in the playroom, and out of doors; they responded to her requests, both verbal and nonverbal; they talked and laughed with her and they set limits for her. They introduced her to new activities; they stood

by when she ventured forth on her own and were there when she needed to re-
treat; they acted as a buffer between Debbie and other people. They did all
these things more or less intuitively, certainly not for any conscious, professionally purposeful reason. Indeed they probably did not recognize their
actions as serving an important nursing function; they did, in fact, say that
Debbie required very little "nursing care." But they succeeded in giving to
her perhaps her first opportunity to develop a sustained relationship with
warm and friendly adults—a relationship in which all found satisfaction and
enjoyment. And further, they provided Debbie with some kinds of experiences out of which she could build some rational understanding of the
world and her relation to it.

And then there was Rose R, age two and one-half. She provides an example of the first situation in which the nursing practitioner recognized the
behavioral manifestations of separation anxiety and consciously made an
effort to base her approach on this knowledge. Rose protested against
her separation vehemently. She cried almost continuously the first 12 hours
after admission and ignored, even rejected, the efforts of several nurses to
comfort her. Her rejection of the staff was so complete, in fact, that several of
them began to ignore Rose. But our practitioner decided that she would be on
hand when Rose was able to use her and that she would attempt, in the
meantime, to show the child that this new environment and the people in it
were trustworthy, friendly, and possible to understand. She visited Rose frequently that first day, sometimes just sitting quietly by her bed for a few
minutes. She talked to her from time to time, telling her about the things
going on around her, and she used familiar terms insofar as possible to
explain repeatedly what was happening. The nurse held Rose for brief periods when she was willing, made frequent references to her mother's return, and showed her the door through which her mother would come. But
most of all she kept returning.

Rose did not seem to recognize her the next day but she made her first
response to the nurse's efforts that morning when she put her arms around
the nurse's neck. Rose's behavior pattern during her five-day hospitalization,
was quite close to that described by Bowlby *et al.*, for the stages of protest
and despair, except that she did respond increasingly to the one nurse beginning with that morning. She never called this nurse by name although she
could talk; but she gave unmistakable evidence of recognition when "her"
nurse appeared, in her facial expression and in her body talk, after the
second day. Rose's mother visited as often as she was allowed, and the
nurse spent time with her and Rose as often as she could. She encouraged Mrs.
R to hold Rose and tried to prepare her for possible changes in the child's
behavior on discharge. It would, of course, be impossible to say at this point

exactly what effect, if any, the nurse's behavior had with respect to the meaning and significance of this short separation experience for Rose. Partial contact with the mother was maintained, and Rose's previous relationship with her appeared to have been a happy one. But because this less dramatic picture of maternal deprivation occurs so frequently in the hospitalization of children, it is perhaps the most important example cited. This is the kind of situation that should draw our first attention and concentrated efforts.

The specific nursing practices suggested in the foregoing examples can be summarized as follows: 1) continuity in contact of a limited number of nursing personnel with the child; 2) genuine interest and involvement by these personnel in the child's current experiences; 3) frequent body contacts; 4) provision for variation in sensory stimulation of the child, including that occurring in the context of social interaction; and 5) establishment of the nurse as a bridge between mother and child. Obviously these practices, as well as others that may be implied, required systematic study if greater certainty about their value and effectiveness is to replace impression. Of these, genuine interest and involvement and the establishment of a bridge are perhaps the most difficult to specify and to measure. Genuine interest and involvement cannot be "legislated." The other factors, which are reasonably concrete, can be observed and recorded either for scientific study or for clinical evaluation. If our notion is correct that the factors which suggest these practices are related to maternal deprivation, then the use of such practices should hold promise in the nursing management of this phenomenon.

• • •

You may ask why the mother has been considered so little in this presentation. This neglect was purposeful, not because continuance of the mother-child relationship during the child's hospitalization is considered of so little importance, but because it is realistic to assume that some separation will continue to occur in most instances in our culture. Further, John A. Rose and Myer Sonis (*American Journal of Psychiatry 116,* Nov. 1959), have suggested that in the presence of a prior-disturbed relationship between mother and child, temporary separation from the real mother may be desirable, although they do not imply that the function this relationship serves for the child should be ignored.

Maternal deprivation and separation anxiety are problems of direct concern to nursing and to nurses. While we must not delude ourselves into thinking that we can be all things to all people, we must search the knowledge available to us in this and other areas for implications for nursing practice. We must then subject these practices to empirical testing insofar as we are able. I have attempted here to present some ideas in one area.

Only further analysis and testing will reveal whether the practices suggested are sound with respect to their anticipated consequences. We do know that nurses must be prepared in knowledge and in skill to fulfill, to the degree possible, functions served by the mother in the mother-child relationship when this relationship must be broken through hospitalization. In addition, we must be prepared to use this knowledge to develop nursing practices which will contribute to the support of that family structure and function which will best serve our society.

41.
Responsibilities to Our Aged

by Alvin I. Goldfarb

Certain present-day concepts of compassion, conscience, and care must be revised if we are to fulfill our individual and social responsibilities to our aged fellowmen.

There are obstructive beliefs which appear to be compassionate that can be summarized in a seemingly well-meaning statement: The aged are rejected and neglected by our society which is youth oriented and discriminates against them; they are discarded by callous families and are relegated to loneliness and discomfort; they are dumped into state hospitals, where they may die of humiliation and the depression that comes from rejection; those who survive must remain because they have no place to go; the young of our society show a lack of admirable character and estimable virtue—they make one wonder how it is "that while one parent could take care of 12 children, 12 children cannot take care of one parent."

This statement purports to exhort us to give better care to the aged. Actually, it does the opposite. It blocks us from effective social action by misstating the facts. It points away from social organization and effort, back to individual and family responsibility, which cannot be realized. To thrust the burden of care of the sick and aged on families can deplete them of time and energy and impoverish them as well.

There are now in this country nearly 20 million persons 65 years of age or older. This represents an increase of older persons from about 3 percent of the population in 1900 to about 10 percent in 1963. The increase is not

Reprinted, with permission, from *The American Journal of Nursing*, LXIV, November 1964, 78–82.

so much because we have been able to prolong life in the already aged as it is because of the decrease of the death rate in infancy, childhood, and youth, and because our population has been augmented by immigration. We have been able to do little to improve the outlook for life in persons 55 and over.

To me, this suggests that persons who in 1900 could survive to be 55 years old had passed critical danger points and had demonstrated specific fitness to survive and, in this decade, persons who have been assisted to live to this age include many whose crises have merely been delayed, so that they may require highly favorable circumstances for further prolongation of life.

To make this clear, we may be helped by reviewing the characteristics of some of the aged who require or can use our medical assistance and to estimate their numbers.

As a group, the aged are poor. About a fifth of them live alone or with nonrelatives, on an income under $940 a year. Those living with families have an income averaging $2,670, which includes contributions from the younger members of the family.

About 6 percent (one million) of them are in institutions. A large number are in public mental hospitals and comprise from 25 to 30 percent of such patients. Half of them have aged in the hospital with conditions of onset in youth or middle age, but the other half are those who were admitted in old age and who have survived. An equivalent number live in nursing homes or old age homes. Many of the aged in mental hospitals have physical functional impairment or illness and need general medical and nursing care. Chronic conditions limit the mobility of 30 percent of all of those 75 and over wherever they are. The average nursing home patient is 80 and may be bedridden and mentally confused. His needs for psychiatric care are so great that a large group of these patients are indistinguishable from many of those in the psychiatric hospitals.

We know that many of the aged who are in their own homes need medical and psychiatric attention. The public health nursing case load indicates the aged at home constitute a massive problem of medical and nursing care. For example, in 1963, aged persons constituted 28 percent of the cases of the Visiting Nurse Service of New York and accounted for 53 percent of the visits made.

In our communities, many aged persons with need for care still go unrecognized. A sampling of housing project residents revealed that 15 percent or more had brain syndrome of at least mild degree, and feelings of insecurity about the ready availability of medical care were even more common. Day centers which serve the aged report many problems of need for medical or psychiatric attention even though their membership is ambulatory and in relatively good general health.

In addition to these clear indications of the extent of need, the statistics on accident, homicide, and suicide rates in old age suggest that there are conditions that lead to death that may be preventable.

At present, although medicine has made many contributions to longevity, added years appear to be more the result of social, economic, and related public health advances, than of the specific individual ministrations of doctor or nurse to patient. Even the excellence and availability of medical care can be considered a social factor, and it is a paradox that making medical care unnecessary has probably contributed most to long life and to the large number of aged.

As doctors and nurses, we must be willing to recognize that the socioeconomic, cultural, and public health developments of the past 60 years which have contributed to the high absolute and relative number of aged now need further development, in response to the new conditions posed by the changed population for which they are largely responsible.

The necessary developments and modifications in our social organization which are important in helping the aged can be considered under the headings of "compassion, conscience, and care." Unfortunately, the technological improvements and socioeconomic developments which have been beneficial may not have been accompanied by revision of personal attitudes, necessary if technical change and progress is to remain beneficial with respect to health and longevity. We are proud that we value human life so much that we preserve the physically sick, the mentally ill, and the debilitated aged. We believe that people should be compassionate and try to rear children so that they try to help or at least do not harm others. We try to train them toward feelings of friendliness and helpfulness to others. But, in a complex society, acculturation toward cooperation can fail or even promote the converse of its aim. Attitudes of kindness, promoted for their beneficial effect on society, may instead result in timidity in providing the protection and supervision our aged need for their health and comfort.

The thought that an overabundance of seemingly loving attitudes may obstruct rather than facilitate the welfare of the aged and of their families surprises many persons.

By mistaking an inflexible sense of obligation for love or compassion, punctilious submission to regulation for conscience, and the preservation of socially obsolete family circles for care and caring, we may block action for the provision of effective care. By overvaluing the role of the family and of friends, and by undervaluing the importance of good institutions, by overestimating the capacities of the family, and by underestimating the need for the development and improvement of social organization, we may promote or perpetuate distress in the aged and their families with wide deleterious social ramifications.

This listing of persons—institutionalized, hospitalized, suicides, accident victims, charges of public health nurses or other agencies, family care burdens, seekers for day centers, old age clubs, and special residences—suggests the needs of the aged for care and their probable subjective emotional and psychological state. Devoted families alone cannot cope with these problems or provide adequate care for their medicalpsychiatric conditions. Individuals who with aging move away from economic, social, and physical self-sufficiency may be in need of considerable psychological and emotional support.

All these factors—psychological, physical, social, and economic—appear to be interrelated. Psychological and emotional disturbance in the aged appears to be more closely associated with physical functional status than with chronological age, and depressive states or low morale more clearly with socioeconomic status than with age or even the actual state of health. Physical status, in turn, appears to be related to prior economic condition and social opportunities.

With relative affluence, the individual has economic security and physical security, which have the protective effect of permitting him to feel relatively free from fear and anger and free to be assertive so that he has limited need for family and friends. Similarly, with a high educational level, he can be expected to have well-established mechanisms of effective psychological, social, and emotional adjustment. When these are well automatized and goal directed, the individual will have self-confidence, self-esteem, purposefulness, and a sense of identity which makes him responsive to the needs of his family and capable of relatively solitary self-enjoyment.

We aim to make our aged patients as self-sufficient as possible in all areas of functioning. In the physical, financial, and social areas, we can expect some increase in self-reliance with our assistance; but in the areas of psychological and emotional functioning we cannot expect to reverse their dependent needs.

Persons who have had good early opportunities usually have had the best chance of internalizing the values of our culture, so that they are capable of playing the various roles required by their achieved or ascribed states as they age and change, or their environment changes about them. They have been and can remain rational, considerate, cooperative, relatively self-reliant, self-disciplined persons, who can gain pleasure through their own efforts and with others. But even persons with good early opportunities can, in our society, age in such a way that each loss, each change in self, and each cultural shift reveals them to be psychologically and emotionally "dependent" as well as socially, economically, or physically in need of aid or support. This dependence is a propensity, with the advent of real or felt helplessness, to seek aid or support in a special way. Either openly or in ways masked from themselves and from others, which can be recognized by the symbolism and trend of their verbal productions or general behavior, they seek to gain, hold, and control others, so they can feel secure, content, and worthwhile. In such persons, the display of need for others, and the subjective feelings of loneliness, boredom, and need for proof of worth through the eyes of others are evidence of their socialization as persons whose self-esteem, self-confidence, and sense of purpose is contingent on their ability, the mastery of special techniques, to gain and hold others.

CONTRIBUTORS TO HIGH MORALE

Factor	Protective Device	Protective Effect	Result
Relative Affluence	Economic security food, shelter, services mobility, medical care	Freedom from fear and anger	Limited need for family and friends
	Physical security power physical comfort pleasure	Assertiveness	
High Educational Level	Well established mechanisms of: psychological, social and emotional adjustment	Self-confidence Self-esteem Self-direction: interests purpose (Sense of identity)	Responsiveness to needs of family
	Diversity and range of interests		
Social Status	Social security	Social independence	Capacity for solitary self-enjoyment
Good Health	Power Mobility Physical comfort or pleasure Physical security	Physical independence	Ability for independent productive or pleasurable activity

What do we expect the nurse to do for the various types of aged persons seen in so many different community or institutional settings? All patients, whatever their condition and wherever they are cared for, may benefit from an approach, attitude, or special use of herself. This approach or use of herself with the patient is determined by the knowledge that patients want to believe that the nurse regards them as of importance, that she has regard for them as persons, that while she takes care of them, she cares for them.

People forget that what they needed when they were helpless children was material and physical care, and that they felt happy to be valued by others because this promised or seemed to guarantee such care. They often come to value being well regarded as more important than being well cared for. This may lead to the disparagement of good physical care in favor of overvaluation of an approach which augments feelings of worth and appears to promise good care and a secure personal relationship. In our efforts to provide the good care, we may tend to forget their "emotional" needs.

Patients want to feel befriended—within their own definition of, or capacity to recognize, friendly relationships. For some this is a gentle, pleasant association. Others, if they are to feel well thought of and secure, may want to believe that the nurse is a somewhat brusque, demanding, or commanding person. The patients generally provide the clues to what they want. Fortunately, the nurse generally need not act out a special part or role, but should rather simply avoid destroying the concept of her that the patient requires. Nurses who need to feel needed, who are frightened by the flattery, ingratiation, or tender feelings of their patients, or who take angry outbursts personally, are at first troubled by the attitudes of their patients. Nurses may need some special training to help them recognize the patient's tendencies to delegate them to a position of quasiparental importance and to accept the delegation gracefully, without trying to convert it into a relationship that fulfills their own needs to feel secure and cared for. They may need opportunities to discuss the parental nurse-patient relationship established by some patients, with specially trained supervisors or even psychiatrists, as in psychiatric hospitals, and old age and nursing homes.

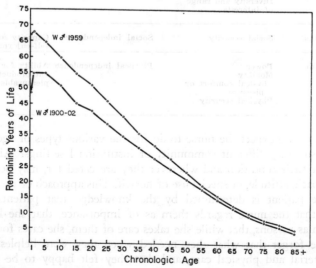

Average number of years of life remaining at stated ages, 1959 &
1900–02, for white males

When the patient feels the nurse is an instrument for his well-being, when she has been accepted as guaranteeing support and aid, the nurse can use the relationship to benefit the patient psychologically and emotionally. The patient's habits or patterns of dealing with others, his social adjustment, can be improved, his "internal" methods of dealing with his own problem can be improved. He can be assisted to differentiate unreasonable fears from possible real dangers, and his wishes from what probably will occur.

The nurse helps the patient—usually slowly—toward rational behavior by decreasing his fear and anger, by favoring an increase in his self-esteem and self-confidence, and by providing him with a sense of purpose in the development of the personal relationship. Her interest, and the interest of her agency or institution in his health, activity, and reactions become the focus of the patient's interest. In his eagerness to ingratiate himself, he becomes interested in himself, in his health, in his activity, and in his reactions. Self-approving interest in himself leads to self-help, to success, and to continued efforts with the development of some actual self-reliance. The nurse is interested in the patient's health and he, to please her, becomes interested in his own health. He tries to follow the regimes which she recommends.

Conversely, he may be obstructive or recalcitrant and attempt to perpetuate symptoms because of his need for her. A recognition of this may assist the nurse to reassure him that improvement will not decrease her interest in him or mean he loses her—although she knows that at some point he may have to do without her. It is our hope that by that time he will no longer need her in person and can relinquish her visits, feeling fully supported and reassured by the recollection of her interest and by the belief that she is personally interested in him and will be readily available should he have need of her. As he succeeds in achieving for himself what he regards as the nurse's goal, he develops self-confidence and in this process he develops purpose, a feeling that life has meaning, that life has continuity. He re-establishes some sense of identity. Never to be forgotten is that the patient's self-reliance develops within the context of a dependent relationship with the nurse. This should not be assaulted. The patient must be permitted to be dependent if he is to become or remain self-reliant.

The acceptance and continuation of dependent relationships with patients is usually to be encouraged, not discouraged, because the preponderance of our population is socialized as dependent and must be permitted to live out a life cycle as dependent persons.

The healthy appear to have been socialized so that they internalized the values of their culture. Each had made an adequate, useful identification with a parental figure or a suitable idealized image, and has been and remains suitably self-assertive, with a capacity to maintain self-esteem through achievement or recollection of success, with self-confidence and sense of purpose. These may be the happier and better adjusted aged.

Unhappy, discontented older persons appear to have been socialized as dependent persons who are anxious when they are, or feel they are, alone, who are prone to accessions of feelings of helplessness and tend to devote their lives to searching for the support of others through whom they gain their sense of worth, their self-confidence, demands on the views of others, and they find purpose in the pursuit of others.

FROM SELF-SUFFICIENCY TO OVERT DEPENDENCY WITH AGING

Factor	Self-Sufficiency ←————————————————→					Overt Dependency
Economic	Wages Pension OASI	Dividends Interest Savings	Insurance	Contribution from Children	Help from extended family or friends	MAA-OA
Social	Friends and Spouse	Family	Neighbors and Community	Special Clubs	Day Centers	Institutio
Physical and/or	Self	Spouse	Children	Old Age Home	Nursing Home	State Hospital
Psychological	Discriminatory Capacity	Well Established Mechanisms of Psychological Adaptation	Well Established Mechanisms of Social and of Emotional Adaptation	Family ———— Friends ———— Companions or Attendants ———— Nurses and Physicians		

They are, with a life cycle of dependency as children, adults, and aged, life-long dependent persons, not regressed when they display their special patterns of appeal, but distressed and signaling their pain. They can be assisted toward self-reliance within their own personality structure, and modes of establishing dependent types of personal relationships. To try to force them toward a nondependent way of functioning is misguided zeal based, I believe, on mistaken, even mythical, notions of personality structure and, in our culture, of the types of personal relationships that are common to our society. These notions of personality structure are more suitable for exhortation and inspiration toward mythical "independence" than as a basis for professional action. I think it is ultraconservative to think of the ill aged as potential workers, as self-reliant members of the general community, as companions and teachers for the young, or as members of a "happy-happy" society of senior citizens. Such goals may be suitable for a certain few chronologically aged persons. Such plans may be an inspirational way to encourage the development of attitudes which lead to individual effort, and at times to supportive self-confidence and to self-esteem, but they do not provide us with solutions for the sick, the poor, and the constitutionally or socially deprived who, having begun with little, tend to end up with less.

In all this, the point which cannot be overemphasized is that in our society, at the present time, to succeed in mobilizing the aged patient toward greater physical self-sufficiency it is almost invariably necessary to permit him to demonstrate or exaggerate his modes of expressing psychological or emotional dependency. He must be permitted to form an emotionally dependent relationship with the nurse. Usually, only this encourages physical mobilization toward greater physical self-sufficiency which her technical know-how implements. Where this does not occur and invalidism persists as a means of holding the nurse, it is helpful to understand the tendency of the patient to exaggerate, utilize, and to exploit physical or mental symptoms to manipulate others. The manipulation is based on helplessness.

Space does not permit a complete discussion of this; there is space merely to reiterate that the dependency needs, the feelings of helplessness of the patient and his search for aid and support from others, which appear to be an obstruction to his improvement and often provoke contempt or anger, are actually aids that can be and should be used for his benefit. Their existence should be gratefully recognized.

42.
A Patient's Concern with Death

by Joan M. Baker and Karen C. Sorensen

On your busy morning rounds, you stop by Mr. Jones' bed. He reaches for your hand and, as he takes it, says, "Nurse, I know I'm dying. Will it be today?"

Mr. Jones has been critically ill and appears exhausted. He looks directly at you, and the silence that follows his question suddenly becomes painful. Should you discuss this with him or remain silent? How can you help Mr. Jones? What could you say? Many questions flash across your mind as the silence continues and Mr. Jones awaits your answer.

Reprinted, with permission, from *The American Journal of Nursing, LXIII,* July 1963, 90–92.

In whatever way you decide to respond to Mr. Jones, there are several factors which will influence your decision. One is why you think Mr. Jones asked you this question. In other words, what is your perception of Mr. Jones' behavior? Do you believe he expects you to have an answer? Perhaps you feel that this is his way of letting you know he is afraid and wants to talk about his fear. Maybe you think he is testing you to find out if you will answer the same as others. Just what does he expect of you?

Other factors which will influence your response to Mr. Jones will be some of your own past experiences related to death and what dying means to you. Maybe talking about death makes you feel sad and inadequate because you have not been able to face and explore your own past experiences related to death. Perhaps to you, death is a personal experience which you feel should not be discussed with others or which should only be discussed with clergymen or doctors. What do you think happens to people when they die?

The nurse realizes that some of her patients may not yet have assigned their own meaning to death, although death may be near. It is important therefore that the discussion should be patient-centered and without the nurse's trying to interject her philosophy into the structure the patient is building. If free discussion is to be maintained, the nurse must not censor ideas which the patient may be presenting.

Many nurses have never pondered and formulated their own ideas about death before being confronted with a question similar to the one asked by Mr. Jones. This indeed is unfortunate and causes many nurses to direct their energies toward helping themselves in the situation rather than the patient.

A person is likely to feel more at ease when he is allowed to explore the meaning that death has for him and to arrive eventually at his own philosophy.

We have pointed out how the nurse's perception of the patient's behavior, combined with her own past experiences and philosophy concerning death, can affect her response to a patient. These factors will determine how the nurse feels when the patient brings up the subject of death. Each nurse will experience a variety of feelings. One nurse's predominant feeling may be confidence in her ability to help the patient communicate effectively about his thoughts and feelings. Another nurse may feel very threatened when the patient brings up such an emotionally charged subject. Thus, she may interfere with the patient's communication while attempting to make herself feel more comfortable.

When a nurse cannot comfortably discuss the subject of death with a patient, she may attempt to terminate the discussion in various ways. Mr. Jones has just asked the nurse if she thinks he will die that day. The nurse might respond by:

1. Moralizing to the patient: "You shouldn't talk that way, Mr. Jones. No one knows when he will die." In effect, this nurse is telling Mr. Jones that it is wrong for him to talk about his death.

2. Stating facts or possible facts which disagree with the feelings the patient is expressing: "I don't think you're going to die today, Mr. Jones. Let me take your pulse. Yes, it's strong and steady and your color is good. This isn't the end of you." This nurse is disregarding the feelings of the patient and using physiological facts to prove to the patient that his concern is not necessary.

3. Denying directly the fact that the patient may die: "No, I don't think you'll die today or even tomorrow." This nurse's response discourages further communication by terminating the discussion with her own opinion.

4. Philosophizing to the patient: "No one really knows what the future holds for him. It is up to each of us to have faith. There will be a tomorrow." Here the nurse states her own philosophy about life and death before giving the patient a chance to formulate his own.

5. Changing the subject: "Who's that in the picture on your night-stand?" This nurse avoids answering the patient and at the same time is showing disrespect for the patient's feelings by ignoring the question.

6. Referring the patient to another person: "I am unable to tell you that. The doctor is better able to tell you what your condition is." Here the nurse is telling the patient that nurses aren't as able to talk with the patient as doctors are.

7. Kidding the patient out of expressing further feelings: "Oh, come on now. You're going to outlive me." This nurse is making light of a very serious matter.

8. Avoiding the question by silence or turning away from the patient. By her silence, the nurse indicates she cannot or will not discuss the matter, and she may busy herself in some activity such as cleaning out a nightstand drawer. (This silence is different from the one in which the nurse is looking at the patient understandingly and encouraging him to go on in the conversation.)

These examples show how a nurse can terminate a conversation and manipulate the patient into a position where his expression of feelings becomes secondary to her own comfort. In many of the examples, the nurse is verbalizing her own ideas instead of exploring those of the patient. In others, she may be prompting the patient to feel guilty about his attempt to talk about death. In all these situations the nurse is saying, "Stop talking about dying." While she may want to help the patient, the nurse's inability to tolerate further discussion may indicate to the patient that she is not interested in him. Such responses force the patient to face this problem alone or to keep seeking for someone who will help him think through his feelings.

How might a nurse participate more effectively with a patient in discussing death? The following situation illustrates some basic principles related to helping the patient communicate his feelings.

Ann Smith is a nurse on the ward where Mr. Jones is a patient. She enters his room and the following interaction takes place:

Mr. J, (weakly), "Oh, hello, Miss Smith." The patient's tone of voice offers the nurse a clue.

Miss S, "Hello, Mr. Jones. I thought I'd drop in for a while and see how you are feeling." The nurse pauses and allows the patient to respond.

Mr. J, "Well, this will probably be your last chance." The patient drops another vague clue.

Miss S, "I don't quite understand what you mean." Instead of jumping to conclusions about what the patient might mean, Miss Smith asks for clarification—she is inviting the patient to speak directly about his concern.

Mr. J, "I'm sinking fast. Do you think I'll die today?" Mr. Jones now speaks directly about his problem and asks the nurse for a direct answer to it.

Miss S, "Why do you ask that, Mr. Jones?" Miss Smith avoids a direct answer to the question and instead invites the patient to express himself further. The nurse stays with the subject rather than terminating it as in the previous examples. The nurse could have been more direct in answering the patient by preceding her comment by, "I don't know, Mr. Jones."

Mr. J, "I'm so weak, I can barely take a drink of water by myself." The patient is just beginning to discuss some of the reasons related to his concern about dying. He waits to see what the nurse will do now.

Miss S, "Yes?" She encourages him to continue—her tone tells him that she is ready to continue listening to him.

Mr. J, "I was pretty sick for a long time. The doctor told my wife that death knocked at my door." Mr. Jones is telling Miss Smith that the doctor implied that death was close at hand.

Miss S, "Yes, I remember." The nurse indicates she is still listening and refrains from making an interpretation.

Mr. J, "I'm glad I didn't go then, but I'm afraid I will now, even though I'm supposed to be better." Mr. Jones is glad to be alive but wonders if he is out of danger.

Miss S, "You're afraid you're going to die now?" Miss Smith, quite sure by now that her patient feels more capable of pursuing the subject, restates in more direct terms what Mr. Jones has said—asking for further elaboration about his feelings.

Mr. J, "Yes. I haven't slept for two nights, I've been so afraid." Patient relates what this fear is doing to hamper his recovery. His statement begins to point out to the nurse some action which will be helpful.

Miss S, "You haven't even been able to sleep?" Again, the nurse reflects on the patient's comment.

Mr. J, "No. I'm afraid I'm going to die. You know, Mother used to say that we each have an angel and when we die this angel goes with us." Mr. Jones again restates his fear and tells the nurse of an idea he has heard about dying.

Miss S, "Oh?" The nurse refrains from commenting directly on this idea.

Mr. J, "Do you think she was right?" (Looks intently at Miss Smith.) The patient is now asking the nurse to be more direct and to communicate her ideas to him.

Miss S (ponderingly), "Well, I don't know, Mr. Jones. What do you think about it?" While Miss Smith responds directly, she remains noncommittal and helps Mr. Jones to explore his ideas further. (Miss Smith realized that what she thought about Mr. Jones' idea was not important, but what was important, was to continue to express interest in the idea and to allow the patient to explore his feelings.)

Mr. J, "I think maybe she was but I'm so tired, I can hardly talk or think about it." Mr. Jones indicates that he, too, believes in the idea he presented as his mother's. He feels too tired to talk further.

Miss S, "Would you feel safer in going to sleep if I stayed with you for a while?" Miss Smith, taking advantage of the information the patient has given her, suggests a therapeutic nursing action.

Mr. J, "You mean sit right by my bed?" He asks for further clarification and indicates a need for closeness.

Miss S, "Yes." Miss Smith recognizes this need and together they have planned the nursing action.

Mr. J, "I think I'll try it." (He turns on his side.) "I don't feel so afraid when someone is with me." Mr. Jones accepts the nursing action and indicates his fear has subsided somewhat.

Three principles have been formulated from the previous interaction. It is hoped, they may lead to helpful therapeutic action in situations where a patient shows concern about death. These principles are not only applicable to discussing death, but may also be used in situations where the patient is attempting to investigate other emotionally charged areas.

1. Don't close the door with your own doubts or fears.

When the patient expresses an idea or opinion and the nurse explores this by asking him for clarification, by asking for more information, and by reflecting back the patient's idea or opinion, and does not state her own, then the patient is allowed a greater degree of freedom in expressing himself and has more opportunity to explore, clarify, and define his own thinking.

However, when the nurse states her own views about what the patient has expressed, which either support or oppose the idea or opinion of the patient, then there will be less opportunity for the patient to explore freely, clarify, and define his own thinking.

2. Lead the patient but don't drag him.

When a patient is vague in his communication, the nurse can help him communicate more clearly and directly by asking the patient what he means, summarizing what she thinks the patient means and asking the patient to validate her summary, or by indicating her own lack of understanding of the patient's communication.

However, when the nurse responds as if she knew what the patient was attempting to communicate, communication may remain vague, distorted, and incomplete.

3. Find a mutual goal.

When the nurse and patient pursue the same goal, or attempt to solve the same problem, it is more likely that the goal will be attained or the problem solved to their mutual satisfaction.

However, when the nurse and patient are pursuing separate goals or problems, blocking and conflict may often be the outcome with resulting mutual dissatisfaction.

The Reverend Peter S. Raible of the University Unitarian Church in Seattle said in a sermon on the theology of death, "In an age when death is so assiduously avoided it is perhaps natural that many are allowed to end their lives in ignorance of what is happening to them or, even more likely, in a sham pretense carried on by relative, patient, and physician alike that death is not at hand."

Nurses, too, are guilty of these offenses. Death is but one phase of life; it is the experience which all of us are destined for from birth. Nurses are becoming increasingly skilled in helping people discuss and meet all phases of life's progression—birth, childhood, adolescence, adulthood, aging. Death—the next phase in the natural progression of life—is too often avoided as a topic of discussion.

We deal physically with the dying and the dead, but do not give the living the natural opportunity to discuss this experience adequately. We need to become more alert to what the patient is saying. Patients may bring up the subject of death in various ways. Let them have the opportunity to express themselves without censure.

Often nurses express concern about harming patients if they discuss death with them. Nurses also express insecurity about exploring this area because they may be asked unanswerable questions. We need to recognize when patients are indicating a desire to explore and also to realize that we cannot give omniscient answers to questions concerning death. Instead, nurses can help each patient formulate his own philosophy of death by keeping their responses free from personal prejudices. We must always keep in mind that some persons may not wish to discuss the subject of death even when its presence is imminent. That is each person's prerogative.

The difficult part of death is not the act of dying itself, we believe, but in preparing for coming death. There are no magic words or pat routines by which one person can help another to adjust to dying. Rather each occasion calls for a personal assessment and decision by the person in the position to help.

INDEX